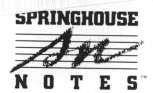

SPRINGHOUSE

NOTES™

NURSING RESEARCH

=== SECOND EDITION ===

Veta H. Massey, RN, PhD
Professor and Chair, Department of Nursing
Brenan University
Gainesville, Georgia

Springhouse Corporation
Springhouse, Pennsylvania

Staff

Executive Director, Editorial
Stanley Loeb

Senior Publisher, Trade and Textbooks
Minnie B. Rose, RN, BSN, MEd

Art Director
John Hubbard

Clinical Consultants
Maryann Foley, RN, BSN; Patricia Kardish Fischer, RN, BSN

Editors
David Moreau, Diane Labus, Janice Fisher

Copy Editors
Diane M. Armento, Debra Davis, Pamela Wingrod

Designers
Stephanie Peters (associate art director),
Jacalyn Facciolo (book designer)

Typography
Diane Paluba (manager), Elizabeth Bergman, Joyce Rossi Biletz, Phyllis Marron, Robin Mayer, Valerie L. Rosenberger

Manufacturing
Deborah Meiris (director), Anna Brindisi, Kate Davis, T.A. Landis

Editorial Assistants
Caroline Lemoine, Louise Quinn, Betsy K. Snyder

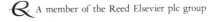 A member of the Reed Elsevier plc group

Library of Congress Cataloging-in-Publication Data

Massey, Veta H.
  Nursing research / Veta H. Massey. — 2nd ed.
    p. cm. — (Springhouse notes)
  Includes bibliographical references and index.
    1. Nursing—research. I. Title. II. Series.
    [DNLM: 1. Nursing Research WY 20.5
M416n 1995]
RT81.5.M28   1995
610.73'072—dc20
DNLM/DLC   94-29595
ISBN 0-87434-742-4   CIP

Contents

Advisory Board and Reviewers

REVIEWERS

1st Edition

Mary Ann Lubno, RN, PhD, CNAA

Associate Dean of the Undergraduate Program
Texas Tech University Health Sciences Center
School of Nursing
Lubbock, Texas

2nd Edition

Angela P. Clark, RN, PhD, FAAN

Associate Professor and Division Chair of Adult Health Nursing
Assistant Dean for Academic Programs
University of Texas at Austin School of Nursing
Austin, Texas

How to Use Springhouse Notes

Springhouse Notes is a multi-volume study guide series developed especially for nursing students. Each volume provides essential course material in an outline format, enabling the student to review the information efficiently.

Special features recur throughout the book to make the information accessible and easy to remember. *Learning objectives* begin each chapter, encouraging the student to evaluate knowledge before and after study. Next, within the outlined text, *key points* are highlighted in shaded blocks to facilitate a quick review of critical information. Key points may include cardinal signs and symptoms, current theories, important steps in a nursing procedure, critical assessment findings, crucial nursing interventions, or successful therapies and treatments. *Points to remember* summarize each chapter's major themes. *Study questions* then offer another opportunity to review material and assess knowledge gained before moving on to new information. Difficult, frequently used, or sometimes misunderstood terms (indicated by small capital letters in the outline) are gathered at the end of each chapter and defined in the *glossary*, Appendix A; answers to the study questions appear in Appendix B.

The Springhouse Notes volumes are designed as learning tools, not as primary information sources. When read conscientiously as a supplement to class attendance and textbook reading, Springhouse Notes can enhance understanding and help improve test scores and final grades.

CHAPTER 1

Introduction to Nursing Research

Learning objectives

Check off the following items once you've mastered them:

☐ Describe the goals of nursing research.

☐ Identify the sources of nursing knowledge.

☐ Discuss the evolution of nursing research over the last century and the implications for future nursing research.

☐ List the major steps in performing research.

☐ Identify the responsibilities that nurses, depending on their education, may be expected to assume in research.

I. Overview of nursing research

A. The primary goal of nursing RESEARCH is to develop a specialized, scientifically based body of knowledge unique to nursing

B. Nursing research has other goals as well
1. Developing and testing nursing theories
2. Providing an understanding of phenomena related to nursing
3. Fostering professional commitment and accountability
4. Helping nurses to make informed decisions in the delivery of patient care
5. Validating the effectiveness of particular nursing measures
6. Helping to document nursing's unique role in health care delivery
7. Improving the quality of care and care delivery
8. Providing a link between theory and practice
9. Advancing nursing as a profession

C. Nursing research that uses the *scientific method* is one of the primary sources of nursing knowledge

D. The scientific method is a systematic approach to solving problems
1. It controls variables and biases
2. It uses EMPIRICAL EVIDENCE to generate generalizable results

E. Researchers use the scientific method primarily for five tasks
1. Describing phenomena
2. Exploring the relationships among phenomena
3. Explaining phenomena and increasing understanding
4. Predicting the causes of and relationships among phenomena
5. Controlling phenomena

F. Basing nursing research on the scientific method is limiting
1. Every research study has flaws
2. No single study proves or disproves a hypothesis
3. Ethical issues can constrain researchers
4. Holistic studies of humans are difficult
5. Adequate control is hard to maintain in a study

G. Nursing knowledge also relies on six other sources
1. Tradition
2. Authority
3. Intuition
4. Trial and error
5. Personal experience
6. Logical reasoning (INDUCTIVE or DEDUCTIVE)

H. Nursing research can be basic or applied
1. *Basic* research
   a. Undertaken to advance knowledge in a given area
   b. Helps the researcher to understand relationships among phenomena

2. *Applied* research
    a. Undertaken to remedy a particular problem or modify a situation
    b. Helps the researcher to make decisions or evaluate techniques

I. Nursing research can be quantitative or qualitative
    1. Quantitative research examines specific phenomena
    2. Qualitative research explores human experiences as they are lived

II. Historical perspective

A. 1850 to 1949
    1. Attempts at nursing research began in the 1850s with Florence Nightingale
        a. She emphasized the importance of systematic observation, data collection, environmental factors, and statistical analyses
        b. Nightingale's research led to attitudinal and organizational changes for nursing and society at large
    2. Research in the early 1900s focused mainly on nursing education; however, case studies on nursing interventions were also conducted in the late 1920s and 1930s, the results of which were published in the *American Journal of Nursing*
    3. The Goldmark Report of 1923, a comprehensive study of nursing education, recommended reorganizing the nursing education system and incorporating it into the university setting
    4. The Brown Report of 1948, which recommended further analysis of nursing functions and nurses' relationships with patients, led to a system for classifying and accrediting nursing schools

B. 1950 to 1959
    1. During the 1950s, research mainly studied nursing activities
    2. Research courses were introduced into baccalaureate-degree nursing programs, and more research courses were added at the master's-degree level
    3. *Nursing Research* began publication in 1952
    4. The American Nurses' Foundation was chartered in 1955 to help the growing number of nurses with advanced education to fund and conduct nursing research
    5. The first nursing unit for clinical practice–oriented research was established in 1957 at the Walter Reed Army Institute of Research

C. 1960 to 1969
    1. During the 1960s, research focused primarily on clinical studies
    2. The American Nurses Association (ANA) sponsored the first nursing research conference aimed at disseminating research findings in 1965
    3. In 1968, nursing archives for historical research were established at Boston University
    4. Nursing studies began to explore theoretical and conceptual frameworks as a basis for practice

D. 1970 to 1979
1. During the 1970s, research focused mainly on improving patient care
2. The ANA established the Commission on Nursing Research in 1972 to facilitate the exchange of ideas among researchers and to recognize excellence in research
3. Additional research journals, such as *Advances in Nursing Science* (1978), *Research in Nursing and Health* (1978), and *Western Journal of Nursing Research* (1979), began publication
4. The National League for Nursing began to consider research a necessary component in the accreditation of nursing education programs

E. 1980 to 1989
1. In the 1980s, interest in qualitative nursing research grew
2. The number of doctoral-level nursing programs and students increased, resulting in increased research
3. The ANA created the Center for Research for Nursing in 1983 to develop reliable data for the profession
4. The National Center for Nursing Research was established within the National Institutes of Health in 1985, putting nursing research into the mainstream of health research activities

F. 1990 to the present
1. The 1990s have seen an increase in integrative reviews and meta-analyses
2. The Agency for Health Care Policy and Research of the U.S. Department of Health and Human Services' Public Health Service developed clinical practice guidelines based on research
3. In 1993, the National Center for Nursing Research was renamed the National Institute for Nursing Research, putting nursing research on the same level as other health-related research
4. Sigma Theta Tau established the Virginia Henderson International Nursing Library, an electronic library making information accessible to researchers worldwide
5. The first electronic nursing journal, the *Online Journal of Knowledge Synthesis for Nursing*, was established in 1993 and publishes critical reviews of research literature

G. Priorities for future nursing research
1. Promoting health and self-care among all groups
2. Preventing behaviorally and environmentally induced health problems
3. Minimizing the negative effects of new health technologies
4. Ensuring that the health needs of vulnerable groups, such as elderly patients and children, are met in effective and acceptable ways
5. Classifying nursing practice phenomena
6. Ensuring that nursing research is guided by ethical principles

7. Developing reliable and valid research instruments to measure outcomes
8. Developing methodologies for the holistic study of humans
9. Designing and evaluating alternative models for health care delivery
10. Evaluating the effectiveness of alternative approaches to nursing education to ensure that practice requirements are met
11. Identifying and analyzing factors that influence nurses' involvement in health policy development
12. Continuing to develop and test nursing theories
13. Replicating studies to gain more confidence in nursing actions
14. Determining the cost of nursing services

III. Steps in performing research

A. General information
  1. A research study typically follows a sequence of steps
  2. At each step, the researcher makes decisions that affect the study
  3. Before conducting a major research study, the researcher may perform a PILOT STUDY, which minimizes the possibility of encountering serious difficulties in the major study and obtains information for improving the major study

B. Research problem (see Chapter 3)
  1. The researcher selects a problem that clarifies the focus of the study
  2. The focus moves from a general topic to a specific problem
  3. The researcher culminates by formulating a PROBLEM STATEMENT

C. Literature review (see Chapter 4)
  1. The researcher uses related literature to examine knowledge to date
  2. The literature must be relevant to the concepts (variables) identified in the problem statement
  3. The review helps direct the researcher in designing the study and interpreting the results

D. Conceptual and theoretical frameworks (see Chapter 5)
  1. These provide structure and link components
  2. They provide a context within which the researcher can interpret the study's results

E. Variables and hypotheses (see Chapter 6)
  1. The researcher predicts the study's outcome based on the relationship among the variables
  2. The researcher must specify how the variables are viewed and how they will be measured

F. Research design (see Chapter 7)
  1. The design provides guidelines with which the researcher tests the hypotheses

2. It directs the selection of the POPULATION, sampling technique, and plan for the researcher's data collection and analysis

G. Population and sample (see Chapter 8)
   1. These establish the criteria that the researcher uses to include subjects
   2. They outline how the subjects will be selected

H. Data collection (see Chapter 9)
   1. The collected data provide the researcher with the information needed to answer the research question
   2. How the data are collected can influence the study's outcome
   3. Data should be evaluated according to specific techniques

I. Data analysis (see Chapter 10)
   1. The researcher consolidates and organizes the data to produce findings that can be interpreted
   2. Analysis involves descriptive procedures, statistical techniques, or logical explanations

J. Results and findings (see Chapter 11)
   1. The researcher draws conclusions from the data and makes recommendations for action or further study
   2. The researcher relates the findings to previous research and to the conceptual or theoretical framework
   3. The researcher disseminates the study's findings for use

IV. Nurses' responsibilities in research

A. General information
   1. Any nurse can participate in research and use its findings
   2. In 1981, the ANA developed guidelines to help nursing educators prepare nurses for research, according to their academic level
   3. As educational preparation increases, the researcher's sophistication also increases
   4. Nurses at all academic and professional levels need to critique previously conducted and newly proposed research

B. Responsibilities of graduates from associate-degree nursing programs
   1. Demonstrate awareness of the value of research
   2. Assist in identifying problem areas and data collection

C. Responsibilities of graduates from baccalaureate-degree nursing programs
   1. Read, interpret, and evaluate research reports
   2. Apply research findings to nursing practice
   3. Identify nursing problems for investigation
   4. Share research findings with peers
   5. Participate in research projects

D. Responsibilities of graduates from master's-degree nursing programs
   1. Analyze and reformulate nursing problems so that they can be tested

  2. Provide nursing expertise to help identify research problems and direct research
  3. Conduct scientific investigations
  4. Collaborate, consult, and assist with others in research projects and applying findings

E. Responsibilities of graduates from doctoral-degree nursing programs
  1. Appraise, design, and conduct nursing research
  2. Develop theoretical explanations of nursing phenomena
  3. Develop methods of scientific inquiry
  4. Use analytical and empirical methods to modify or extend knowledge
  5. Provide leadership in promoting nursing research

Points to remember

Nursing research is essential for developing a scientific knowledge base and for advancing nursing as a profession.

Nursing knowledge is derived from the scientific method, tradition, authority, intuition, trial and error, personal experience, and logical reasoning.

Nursing research may be basic or applied, quantitative or qualitative.

Nursing research has been shaped by key historical events.

Research includes sequential steps that provide order and control.

Every nurse, regardless of educational level, has certain responsibilities in the research process.

Glossary

The following terms are defined in Appendix A, page 111.

deductive reasoning   population

empirical evidence   problem statement

inductive reasoning   research

pilot study

Study questions

To evaluate your understanding of this chapter, answer the following questions in the space provided; then compare your responses with the correct answers in Appendix B, page 115.

1. What is the primary goal of nursing research? _____

_____

_____

2. What is the difference between basic research and applied research?

_____

_____

3. What contributions did Florence Nightingale make to nursing research?

_____

_____

4. Why might a researcher conduct a pilot study? _____

_____

_____

5. What is the responsibility of all nurses, regardless of academic or professional level, in research? _____

_____

_____

CHAPTER 2

Ethical Considerations in Nursing Research

Learning objectives

Check off the following items once you've mastered them:

☐ Identify historical events affecting professional guidelines and ethical codes.

☐ Compare and contrast existing professional guidelines and codes for conducting ethical research.

☐ Describe the characteristics and functions of an institutional review board.

☐ List the five human rights that require protection in research, and describe the procedures for protecting those rights.

☐ Outline the major elements of informed consent.

☐ List pertinent questions to ask when critiquing the ethical aspects of a research study.

I. Introduction

A. Nursing research must be ethical in its development and implementation to protect human subjects without compromising the quality of the research

B. Ethics in nursing research involves applying those principles and actions mandated by professional, legal, and social rules to protect human subjects

C. Ethical actions taken by researchers should include four components
   1. Protecting the rights of subjects
   2. Ensuring that a study's potential benefits outweigh its risks to the subjects
   3. Submitting the proposed study for institutional review
   4. Obtaining an INFORMED CONSENT from each subject

II. Historical events affecting ethical research

A. General information
   1. Unethical experiments and mistreatment of human research subjects in early studies prompted the need for ethical conduct in research and led to the development of professional guidelines and ethical codes
   2. Experimental studies noted for unethical treatment of human subjects include Nazi medical experiments, the Tuskegee syphilis study, the Jewish Chronic Disease Hospital study, and the Willowbrook hepatitis study

B. Nazi medical experiments
   1. Conducted from 1933 to 1945 by the Third Reich in Europe to produce a pure German race
   2. Included euthanasia, sterilization, and numerous medical experiments, such as exposing subjects to high altitudes, freezing temperatures, diseases, and untested drugs
   3. Based the selection of subjects on political or religious status (prisoners of war, Jews)
   4. Allowed no opportunity for subjects to refuse participation
   5. Performed to generate knowledge and eliminate "inferior" people

C. Tuskegee syphilis study
   1. Performed in Tuskegee, Alabama, from 1932 to 1972 under the supervision of the U.S. Public Health Service
   2. Conducted to determine the course of syphilis in adult black males
   3. Withheld from the subjects knowledge about the availability of penicillin after it proved to be an effective treatment
   4. Also withheld information about the purpose of the research

D. Jewish Chronic Disease Hospital study
   1. Conducted in 1963 in Brooklyn, New York

    2.   Involved the injection of live cancer cells into 22 patients to determine their rejection responses

    3.   Conducted without the informed consent of the subjects, knowledge of the subjects' physicians, or approval from the hospital research committee

E. Willowbrook hepatitis study
    1.   Conducted during the 1960s and 1970s in Willowbrook, New York
    2.   Used institutionalized, mentally retarded children as subjects
    3.   Inoculated groups of newly institutionalized children with hepatitis viruses to evaluate their responses
    4.   Forced parents to consent by allowing admissions to the research ward only

III. Professional guidelines and codes

A. General information
    1.   Abuse of human subjects by unethical researchers directly influenced the development of ethical codes and guidelines
    2.   Codes and guidelines developed by professional groups to govern ethical behavior and conduct are difficult to formulate because definitions of "right" and "wrong" are typically vague and subjective
    3.   Researchers must consider ethical guidelines continuously during a study to ensure that research is conducted ethically (see *Checklist: Ethical Aspects of Research*)

B. The Nuremberg Code
    1.   Developed in 1949 as a result of unethical experimentation spotlighted during Nazi criminal trials
    2.   Was the first international effort to create formal standards involving human research subjects
    3.   Included guidelines for voluntary consent, subjects' protection from harmful experiments, subjects' right to withdraw from a study, grounds for discontinuing a study, the need for balance between potential risks and potential benefits in a study, and the researcher's necessary qualifications

C. The Declaration of Helsinki
    1.   Adopted in 1964 and revised in 1975 by the World Medical Association
    2.   Based on the Nuremberg Code
    3.   Differentiated therapeutic research, such as research conducted to explore the beneficial effects of a new treatment, from nontherapeutic research aimed toward building a knowledge base
    4.   Identified the importance of qualifying the type of research (therapeutic or nontherapeutic) when explaining potential benefits and risks to prospective subjects
    5.   Stated that subjects must be informed of the personal risks and potential benefits before agreeing to participate

---

CHECKLIST: ETHICAL ASPECTS OF RESEARCH

Use the following questions to critique the ethical aspects of a research study.

	Yes	No
• Was the research approved by an institutional review board or a similar ethical committee?	☐	☐
• Was the researcher qualified to conduct the study?	☐	☐
• Did the study's potential benefits for subjects outweigh the risks?	☐	☐
• Did the researcher take measures to prevent or minimize psychological and physical harm or discomfort to the subjects?	☐	☐
• Were the subjects recruited without coercion?	☐	☐
• Were the subjects told about the potential benefits and risks associated with participation?	☐	☐
• Did the researcher disclose sources of funding?	☐	☐
• Were the study's purposes and procedures fully explained in advance to the subjects?	☐	☐
• Did the researcher obtain informed consent from all participating subjects?	☐	☐
• Did all subjects have an opportunity to decline participation before and during the study?	☐	☐
• If vulnerable subjects were used, was their inclusion necessary?	☐	☐
• Was each subject's right to privacy and anonymity protected?	☐	☐
• Did the researcher maintain objectivity when reporting the findings?	☐	☐
• Did the researcher credit others who assisted with the study?	☐	☐

---

    6. Emphasized the importance of subjects' written consent

D. American Nurses Association Human Rights Guidelines
    1. Developed in 1968 and revised in 1975 and 1985 as specific guidelines for nursing research
    2. Addressed ethical and practical issues related to clinical research
    3. Outlined the rights of nurses to perform research and to gather information and knowledge necessary to complete research studies
    4. Identified the rights of subjects and nurses involved in research

IV. Federal guidelines for conducting ethical research

A. General information
  1. The Department of Health, Education, and Welfare proposed the first set of regulations for protecting human subjects in 1973
  2. Strict regulations for research involving human subjects were published in May 1974, along with additional regulations for vulnerable populations, such as terminally ill and mentally impaired individuals, children, and persons confined to institutions

B. The Belmont Report
  1. Presented in 1978 by the National Commission for the Protection of Human Subjects
  2. Provided the basis for the development of various protective procedures, such as informed consent
  3. Identified three ethical principles relevant to research
    a. Respect
    b. Beneficence
    c. Justice

C. The National Research Act
  1. The National Research Act of 1974 mandated the use of an INSTITUTIONAL REVIEW BOARD (IRB) for any organization receiving federal funding and performing research with human subjects
  2. IRBs review research studies, ensure the protection of subjects' rights, and report noncompliance by researchers
  3. IRBs are authorized to approve or disapprove proposals, require modifications, or suspend the approval of research; approval of all proposals must meet federal guidelines
  4. Studies demonstrating no apparent risk or only minimal risk to subjects may receive a brief review; studies demonstrating a higher risk receive a full IRB review
  5. A study must receive some form of IRB approval before the researcher can initiate it

V. Protection of human rights

A. General information
  1. Human rights are demands or privileges to which a person is entitled
  2. The main purpose of professional guidelines and ethical codes is to protect human rights
  3. In any study, the researcher must weigh potential benefits and risks
  4. VULNERABLE SUBJECTS, such as hospitalized patients, children, prisoners, or the mentally incompetent, require additional protection of their human rights
  5. Human rights that require protection include the rights to self-determination, privacy, ANONYMITY and CONFIDENTIALITY, fair treatment, and protection from harm

B. Right to self-determination
1. The right to self-determination is a person's right to act independently and make individual decisions
2. This right is protected when the researcher informs the subject of all aspects of a study and allows the subject to choose whether to participate and whether to withdraw from the study at any time without penalty
3. This right is violated if the subject is coerced into participating, becomes a subject without realizing it, or is deceived in any way about the research

C. Right to privacy
1. The right to privacy is an individual's freedom to determine when and how much private information will be shared
2. This right is protected when an informed subject voluntarily shares private information
3. This right is violated when private information is obtained without the subject's knowledge or against the subject's will

D. Right to anonymity and confidentiality
1. The researcher is responsible for keeping obtained information and the subject's identity private
2. Anonymity is maintained if the researcher does not know the subject's identity; confidentiality is ensured if the subject's name is separated from the data
3. This right is protected by analyzing data according to groups and reporting findings so that individual responses cannot be recognized
4. This right is violated when an unauthorized person gains access to personal information
5. Violations of this right may harm the subject and lead to loss of trust in the researcher or research study

E. Right to fair treatment
1. The researcher is responsible for selecting and treating all subjects in the same unbiased manner
2. To ensure fair treatment, the researcher must ensure that subjects know beforehand their expected roles and how the researcher plans to interact in the study
3. This right is protected by random selection of subjects
4. This right is violated when subjects are selected because they are readily available or easily manipulated or because of some other reason unrelated to the study

F. Right to protection from harm
1. The researcher is responsible for protecting the subject from unnecessary discomfort or injury resulting from the study
2. This right is protected by the researcher's attempts to maximize a study's potential benefits and minimize its risks

3. This right is violated when the risks to subjects outweigh the benefits

VI. Informed consent

A. General information
   1. All researchers are required to obtain informed consent from all participating subjects, unless it may influence the outcome
   2. Informed consent (oral or written) implies that subjects have sufficient information, are able to comprehend the information, and have free choice to participate

B. Key elements of an informed consent
   1. The study's purpose
   2. The researcher's qualifications
   3. The population being studied and the reasons for selecting it
   4. A description of how and why the individual was selected for the study
   5. An explanation of the procedures used
   6. The time required for participation
   7. The risks related to participation
   8. The benefits that reasonably can be expected from participation
   9. The alternative procedures, if any, that might benefit the subject
   10. The procedure for maintaining anonymity and confidentiality
   11. The availability of treatments should injury result
   12. The person to contact for answers to questions, concerns about human rights, or follow-up treatment of injuries resulting from the research
   13. The subject's freedom to choose whether to participate or withdraw

Points to remember

The Nazi medical experiments, Tuskegee syphilis study, Jewish Chronic Disease Hospital study, and Willowbrook hepatitis study influenced the development of professional guidelines and ethical codes.

The American Nurses Association Human Rights Guidelines is the only professional code to identify the rights of subjects and nurses involved in research.

Any organization that receives federal funding and performs research with human subjects must have an institutional review board to protect the subjects' rights.

Each human subject has the right to self-determination, privacy, anonymity and confidentiality, fair treatment, and protection from harm.

Children and persons who are terminally ill, mentally impaired, or institutionalized are considered vulnerable subjects and consequently require extra protection.

Glossary

The following terms are defined in Appendix A, page 111.

anonymity

confidentiality

informed consent

institutional review board

vulnerable subject

Study questions

To evaluate your understanding of this chapter, answer the following questions in the space provided; then compare your responses with the correct answers in Appendix B, page 115.

1. Which experimental studies are noted for their unethical treatment of human subjects? _____

    _____

    _____

2. What international code resulted from the unethical experimentation spot lighted during the Nazi criminal trials? _____

    _____

    _____

3. What three ethical principles are relevant to research? _____

    _____

    _____

4. What human rights require protection in ethical research? _____

    _____

    _____

CHAPTER 3

Research Problem Selection

Learning objectives

Check off the following items once you've mastered them:

- ☐ Identify how nurse researchers select and formulate research problems.
- ☐ Describe the information found in the purpose of a study.
- ☐ List four sources for nursing research problems.
- ☐ Describe the factors to consider when selecting a research problem.
- ☐ List pertinent questions to ask when critiquing a research problem statement and purpose.

I. Introduction

A. One of the most important steps in research is selecting the problem and formulating the problem statement and purpose
  1. The researcher selects a topic and narrows it into a specific problem
  2. The problem identifies the area of concern and provides direction for the entire study
  3. The problem guides the study toward a quantitative or qualitative approach
  4. The problem must be stated clearly before it can be solved

B. The ability to wonder about situations helps the researcher identify research problems

C. After deciding *what* to study, the researcher begins formulating *why* to conduct the research

D. The purpose of the study, which typically evolves from the research problem, clarifies a number of issues
  1. The extent of the problem
  2. The significance of the problem
  3. The rationale for the study
  4. The researcher's intentions
  5. The clinical context of the study
  6. The ways in which findings will be used

E. The purpose typically concludes with the problem statement

II. Sources for research problems

A. General information
  1. To identify research problems, the researcher must be aware of personal thoughts, observations, and everyday experiences that signal potential areas of concern
  2. Primary sources for research problems include nursing practice, literature, theory, and interactions with peers and researchers

B. Sources in nursing practice
  1. Questions about patient care
  2. Observations of patient and nurse behaviors
  3. Patient care conferences
  4. Complaints and expressions of dissatisfaction from patients and staff
  5. Current nursing procedures compared with new techniques
  6. Chart reviews

C. Literature sources
  1. Journals and textbooks
  2. Abstracts
  3. THESES and DISSERTATIONS

D. Theory sources
1. The work of nursing theorists
2. Theories developed in other disciplines
3. Personal theories

E. Sources involving interactions with peers and researchers
1. Formal educational experiences
2. Staff-development education and orientation programs
3. Policy and procedure committee meetings
4. Journal clubs

III. Factors to consider when selecting a research problem

A. General information
1. The selection of a research problem is not determined by any specific rules
2. The most important factors to consider are the problem's significance, researchability, feasibility, and interest to the researcher

B. Considerations related to significance
1. Will conducting the study expand nursing's knowledge base?
2. Will conducting the study improve nursing practice or policy?
3. Will conducting the study benefit patients, nurses, or society?

C. Considerations related to researchability
1. The problem should not involve ethical or moral issues
2. All problems should be capable of being defined and measured
3. The problem should be specific enough to be manageable

D. Considerations related to feasibility
1. The study should be able to be completed within the allotted time
2. Willing subjects should be available to participate in the study
3. Sufficient funding, facilities, and equipment should be available
4. The researcher should have the expertise required
5. Co-workers should be available and willing to cooperate
6. No unfair or unethical demands should be imposed

E. Considerations related to researcher's interest
1. Levels of enthusiasm can be expected to rise and fall
2. Unless the problem is especially interesting and appealing, the researcher may find the study too tedious or too difficult to complete

IV. Formulating the problem statement

A. General information
1. The researcher should write the research problem and purpose before beginning the study (see *Checklist: Problem Statement and Purpose,* page 22)

CHECKLIST: PROBLEM STATEMENT AND PURPOSE

Use the following questions to critique the research problem and purpose of a study.

	Yes	No
• Does the researcher describe the problem's significance to nursing?	☐	☐
• Has the researcher outlined the rationale for conducting the study?	☐	☐
• Does the problem statement clearly identify the population and the variables being studied?	☐	☐
• Does the problem statement express a relationship between the variables?	☐	☐
• Does the problem statement suggest empirical testability?	☐	☐
• Has the researcher considered practical issues, such as time, funding, facilities, equipment, and the cooperation of others?	☐	☐

---

    2. Writing the problem statement may help the researcher to pinpoint uncertainties that need clarification before the study can proceed

B. Purposes of the problem statement
    1. To provide direction to the research study
    2. To specify what the researcher will examine
    3. To help any user of the research evaluate the study

C. Items typically included in the problem statement
    1. VARIABLES to be studied and the relationship
    2. Specifics about the population being studied
    3. The possibility of using EMPIRICAL TESTING

D. Forms of the problem statement
    1. The *interrogative* form poses the problem as a question
    2. The *declarative* form expresses the problem as a statement

E. Correlational or comparative statements
    1. A *correlational* statement discusses the possibility of a relationship between the variables
    2. A *comparative* problem statement discusses the possibility of a difference between the variables

F. The problem statement for a qualitative study may simply identify the area of concern requiring study

Points to remember

Selecting a research problem is a key step in the research process.

After the researcher has identified a problem to study, the problem is refined and narrowed to a specific topic.

The purpose of the study should introduce the problem and indicate why it is being researched.

The problem should be significant, researchable, feasible, and interesting to the researcher.

The problem statement should identify the key variables, specify the population being studied, and imply whether empirical testing is possible.

Glossary

The following terms are defined in Appendix A, page 111.

dissertation

empirical testing

thesis

variable

Study questions

To evaluate your understanding of this chapter, answer the following questions in the space provided; then compare your responses with the correct answers in Appendix B, page 115.

1. Why is research problem identification an important step? _____

   _____

   _____

2. What are possible sources for a research problem? _____

   _____

   _____

3. Which factors should be considered when selecting a research problem?

   _____

   _____

4. What two forms might a problem statement take? _____

   _____

   _____

CHAPTER 4

Literature Review

Learning objectives

Check off the following items once you've mastered them:

☐ Explain why a researcher conducts a literature review.

☐ Explain research findings, theoretical information, methodological information, opinion articles, and anecdotal descriptions.

☐ Describe methods for organizing the information and the mechanics of writing the review.

☐ Discuss initial and secondary searches.

☐ Explain how to conduct manual and computer literature searches.

☐ Identify criteria for critiquing a literature review.

I. Introduction

A. In quantitative research, the LITERATURE REVIEW is done at the start and lays the foundation for the research project

✳ B. In qualitative research, the literature review may be done after data are analyzed; the literature is compared and contrasted with the study findings (see Chapters 7 and 10)

C. The researcher conducts the review by thoroughly examining all available scientific and theoretical information related to the research problem
  1. The amount of available literature depends on how well the topic has been researched previously
  2. A short, well-organized review of pertinent studies is more valuable than a long, rambling review of irrelevant studies

D. A thorough review should include primary and secondary sources
  1. PRIMARY SOURCES, containing original research findings, are preferred and should be used whenever possible
  2. SECONDARY SOURCES, containing interpretations of research findings, are helpful in providing bibliographical information

II. Purposes of the review

A. General information
  1. A literature review helps the researcher to gauge what is known and unknown about the research problem
  2. A review can serve many purposes
    a. Help the researcher to identify or refine the research problem
    b. Strengthen the rationale for the research
    c. Develop a conceptual framework for the study
    d. Provide a useful approach to conducting the study
    e. Explain or support the findings

B. Identifying or refining the research problem
  1. Reading clinically related literature may help the researcher to recognize areas that need further research and study
  2. The research problem may be refined during the literature review

C. Strengthening the rationale for the research
  1. A lack of literature related to the problem may indicate that the problem needs further study
  2. Conversely, the researcher may find that the problem has been extensively researched, indicating that another study is unnecessary

D. Developing a conceptual framework for the study
  1. In reviewing the literature, the researcher may discover a theory to serve as an approach to the study
  2. The review may lead the researcher to formulate ideas about how the research problem and concepts are linked

E. Providing a useful approach to conducting the study
   1. The literature review may reveal specific research strategies and procedures used in previous studies
   2. The researcher may be able to adapt an approach used in a previous study or develop a new approach to conducting the research

F. Explaining or supporting the findings
   1. The literature review may reveal findings that are similar to or different from those obtained in the current study
   2. The literature review may be used to verify relationships and theories that emerged from the data obtained in the study

III. Review process

A. General information
   1. The researcher conducts a search or a series of searches to find relevant references
   2. The researcher should pursue as many relevant references as possible when conducting a literature review
   3. The researcher reviews all the available information and decides which references to include in the written review

B. Types of information to review
   1. Research findings from previous related studies
   2. Theoretical information concerning broader problem issues
   3. Methodological information on research methods previously used
   4. Opinion articles discussing specific viewpoints or attitudes about the problem; the researcher should keep in mind their subjectivity and limited use
   5. Anecdotal descriptions of others' experiences; the researcher should keep in mind their limited use

C. Conducting an initial search
   1. In an initial search, the researcher scans pertinent publications, including indexes to nursing and health care literature, bibliographies, ABSTRACTS, and other primary and secondary sources, to develop an overview of knowledge available on the problem
   2. The initial review also helps the researcher to determine whether the problem has already been thoroughly studied, whether necessary instruments and tools are available to measure the variables, and whether ideas and beliefs about the problem are correct
   3. This step enables the researcher to decide whether to proceed with the study

D. Conducting a secondary search
   1. In a secondary search, the researcher makes a concerted effort to review all published information related to the problem

    2. The researcher typically begins by searching for the most recent publications

E. Evaluating the information
    1. All references should be summarized and classified for easy retrieval
    2. Reading the abstract or summary is a reliable way to determine the potential usefulness of an article
    3. The reviewer's notes, typically made on index cards or typed into a computer, should include a synopsis of each article and should be organized according to categories

F. Writing a literature review
    1. Before writing the review, the researcher selects appropriate sources from related literature
        a. The researcher typically selects sources based on their relevance to the problem statement and the study's purpose
        b. The researcher typically organizes the selected sources according to concept, theoretical or research classification, ability to support the study's framework, and ability to explain the study's finding
    2. The researcher typically develops an outline as a guide for writing the introduction, body, and summary of the literature review
    3. The introduction describes the organization and purpose of the review
    4. The body, which contains a detailed analysis of relevant studies, typically focuses on research and theoretical information
    5. In the body, the researcher compares and contrasts studies with similar methodology or results, pointing out consistencies and contradictions while striving for objectivity; the researcher should try to present the studies logically, remembering to relate each study to others and to paraphrase material whenever possible
    6. The summary typically discusses the quality of the literature reviewed, identifies gaps in knowledge, and demonstrates the need for the study (see *Checklist: Literature Review*)

IV. Manual literature search

A. General information
    1. A manual search, which is typically time-consuming but relatively inexpensive, is a hands-on way to locate and review literature
    2. This type of search requires familiarity with the library and various index tools, such as card catalogs, medical and nursing indexes, abstracts, and bibliographies

B. Card catalogs
    1. A card catalog is the main source for locating books in a library
    2. In many libraries, the card catalog is listed on an on-line computer

C. Indexes
    1. Indexes are usually organized according to subject and author

---

CHECKLIST: LITERATURE REVIEW

Use the following questions to critique the literature review portion of a study.

	Yes	No
• Does the literature review immediately follow the introduction and problem statement?	☐	☐
• Are all the major variables included in the review?	☐	☐
• Did the researcher use mostly primary sources?	☐	☐
• Did the review include recent literature?	☐	☐
• Did the researcher include most major studies done on the problem?	☐	☐
• Did the researcher include mostly theoretical or research articles rather than opinion or anecdotal articles?	☐	☐
• Did the researcher include a summary that critically evaluates the literature, identifies gaps, and demonstrates how the current study will fill the gaps?	☐	☐
• Is the review logically organized and objective?	☐	☐

---

  2. Indexes are the main source for locating articles published in journals
  3. A number of indexes are of key importance to nursing researchers
     a. *Cumulative Index to Nursing and Allied Health Literature* includes listings from more than 300 nursing and allied health journals
     b. *International Nursing Index* includes listings on nursing literature from around the world
     c. *Nursing Studies Index* includes listings on nursing literature from 1900 to 1959
     d. *Index Medicus* includes more than 3,000 biomedical journals
     e. *Hospital Literature Index* contains references on health care planning and administration

D. Abstracts (brief synopses of articles)
   1. *Nursing Research Abstracts,* published from 1960 to 1978, in *Nursing Research* journal, contains abstracts of nursing-related studies
   2. *Nursing Abstracts* contains abstracts of significant nursing research studies published since 1979
   3. *Excerpta Medica* includes abstracts from the basic biological sciences
   4. *Dissertation Abstracts International* includes abstracts from doctoral dissertations published throughout the world

E. Bibliographies
   1. Bibliographies contain lists of publications on specific topics
   2. They are included in bibliographical indexes as well as at the end of most research articles, books, theses, and dissertations

V. Computer literature search

A. General information
   1. Computer searches are used to access bibliographic information that has been stored in DATABASES
   2. A computer search can be done at any library that has access to the database; a microcomputer equipped with a modem and communications software also may be used to search many databases
   3. To locate appropriate information, the researcher must narrow the topic and determine key words to use in the search
   4. Cost depends on the database searched and the time spent searching
   5. Advanced technology has made computer searches readily available, comprehensive, and invaluable

B. Databases
   1. *CINAHL (Nursing & Allied Health)* corresponds with the information found in *Cumulative Index to Nursing and Allied Health Literature* from 1983 to the present
   2. *MEDLINE* corresponds with the information found in *Index Medicus, International Nursing Index,* and *Index to Dental Literature* from 1966 to the present
   3. *NTIS* covers all publications found in the *Government Reports Announcements* from 1964 to the present
   4. *HEALTH (Health Planning and Administration)* corresponds with the information found in *Hospital Literature Index* from 1975 to the present
   5. *ERIC* corresponds with the information found in *Resources in Education* and *Research in Education* from 1966 to the present
   6. *Dissertation Abstracts Online* corresponds with the information found in *Dissertation Abstracts International* from 1861 to the present
   7. *CATLINE* contains references for books and serials cataloged at the National Library of Medicine
   8. *BIOETHICSLINE* includes citations from 1973 to the present concerning ethical questions in health care housed at the National Library of Medicine and the Kennedy Institute of Ethics

C. Virginia Henderson International Nursing Library
   1. Sigma Theta Tau established the library to be a computerized collection of databases and knowledge resources
   2. The library contains an on-line network and electronic journal
   3. The electronic databases include Directory of Nurse Researchers; Research Conference Proceedings; Sigma Theta Tau International Grant Recipients and Projects; Information Resources Database; and tables of contents of *IMAGE: Journal of Nursing Scholarship*
   4. Subscribers can also access other services, such as Online Conferencing, and read the Sigma Theta Tau International News

Points to remember

A literature review demonstrates what is known about a research problem and validates the need for the current study.

The types of information reviewed include research findings, theoretical information, methodological information, opinion articles, and anecdotal descriptions.

Notes should be systematically recorded and categorized for easy retrieval of information.

The written literature review should be logically organized and objective and should contain mostly research and theoretical sources.

Sources may be searched manually in card catalogs, indexes, abstracts, and bibliographies or by computer through databases.

Glossary

The following terms are defined in Appendix A, page 111.

abstract

database

literature review

primary source

secondary source

Study questions

To evaluate your understanding of this chapter, answer the following questions in the space provided; then compare your responses with the correct answers in Appendix B, pages 115 and 116.

1. Why does a researcher conduct a literature review? _____

   _____

   _____

2. What purposes might a literature review serve? _____

   _____

   _____

3. What types of literature might the researcher review? _____

   _____

   _____

4. What is the researcher's main source for manually locating articles published in journals?_____

   _____

5. What are the advantages of a computer search over a manual search?

   _____

   _____

CHAPTER 5

Conceptual and Theoretical Frameworks

Learning objectives

Check off the following items once you've mastered them:

☐ Describe the purpose of frameworks in nursing research.

☐ Explain person, environment, health, and nursing as concepts used in nursing research.

☐ Discuss the uses of conceptual and theoretical frameworks.

☐ Identify at least four nursing theories and four theories borrowed from other disciplines that are frequently used to guide nursing research.

☐ List the common problems related to conceptual and theoretical frameworks.

☐ State criteria for critiquing conceptual and theoretical frameworks.

I. Introduction

A. A framework, also called a frame of reference, is the logical but abstract structure of a research study
   1. In quantitative research, the framework is a testable theory
   2. In qualitative research, the framework is a philosophy, and a theory may be developed as an outcome of the study

B. The framework helps the researcher to organize the study and interpret the results
   1. The researcher uses the framework as a guide through the entire research process, beginning with the HYPOTHESIS and ending with the study's conclusions
   2. The researcher organizes and explains all of the information acquired in the study through the framework's context
   3. Working within a framework enables the researcher to link the research to nursing's body of knowledge, allowing the findings to be generalized beyond the specific study

C. All frameworks are based on the identification of key CONCEPTS and the relationships between or among those concepts
   1. Concepts typically are abstract (such as "pain" or "grief"), but they can also be concrete (such as "temperature" or "weight")
   2. The researcher formulates PROPOSITIONS to identify concept relationships

D. Four key concepts — person, environment, health, and nursing — are of particular interest to nursing researchers
   1. *Person,* the recipient of nursing care, may be an individual, a family, or a community
   2. *Environment,* the setting in which nursing occurs, typically revolves around the person's significant others and surroundings
   3. *Health,* the person's state of wellness or illness, is identified as the purpose of nursing
   4. *Nursing,* the actions taken by nurses to benefit the person

E. A framework can derive from related concepts (conceptual) or an existing THEORY (theoretical)
   1. Although the terms conceptual framework and theoretical framework are sometimes used interchangeably, they have different meanings
   2. CONCEPTUAL FRAMEWORKS, usually less formal than theoretical frameworks, are used for studies in which existing theory is inapplicable or insufficient
   3. *Theoretical frameworks,* usually more formal than conceptual frameworks, are used for studies based on existing theories
   4. Conceptual and theoretical frameworks may be represented as models
      a. A MODEL is a symbolic representation that helps to express abstract concepts and relationships easily, using minimal words

b. A model can be represented schematically (using boxes, arrows, or other symbols) or statistically (using letters, numbers, and mathematical symbols)

II. Conceptual frameworks

A. General information
   1. A conceptual framework is derived from empirical observation and intuition
   2. The researcher develops the framework by identifying and clarifying the concepts to be used in the study, then specifying the proposed relationships among the concepts
   3. A conceptual framework may be more global and abstract than a theoretical framework

B. Purposes of conceptual frameworks
   1. To clarify concepts and propose relationships among the concepts
   2. To provide a context for interpreting the study findings
   3. To explain observations
   4. To encourage theory development

C. Uses of conceptual frameworks in nursing
   1. Expanding nursing's knowledge base
   2. Defining nursing
   3. Providing a framework when existing theory is insufficient
   4. Clarifying concepts and the relationships among those concepts
   5. Helping nurses provide patient care

III. Theoretical frameworks

A. General information
   1. A theoretical framework is based on a theory derived from specific concepts and propositions that are induced or deduced
   2. Theories are always invented, never discovered; they can be tested but never proved

B. Purposes of theoretical frameworks
   1. To test theories
   2. To make research findings meaningful and generalizable
   3. To explain observations
   4. To predict and control situations
   5. To stimulate research and expand nursing's knowledge base

C. Uses of theoretical frameworks in nursing
   1. Expanding nursing's knowledge base
   2. Defining nursing
   3. Clarifying concepts
   4. Formulating hypotheses for testing
   5. Helping nurses provide patient care

IV. Conceptual and theoretical frameworks used in nursing research

A. General information
  1. Nursing researchers use conceptual and theoretical frameworks developed by nurses and other professionals
  2. Nursing frameworks create formal explanations of what constitutes the profession of nursing
     a. Nursing frameworks vary in the way they define and link key concepts and in the way they emphasize some relationships over others
     b. Nursing frameworks are relatively new tools still being developed
     c. Researchers need to test nursing frameworks to help formulate and refine nursing theories, making them more useful to nursing practice
  3. Nursing researchers may use frameworks from other disciplines that can be adapted to nursing-related concepts
     a. These disciplines include psychology, sociology, education, physiology, and anthropology
     b. Adapted frameworks are sometimes referred to as borrowed or shared

B. Examples of nursing frameworks
  1. M. Rogers's "Science of Unitary Human Beings"
  2. D. Orem's "Self-Care Model"
  3. C. Roy's "Adaptation Model"
  4. I. King's "Theory of Goal Attainment"
  5. D. Johnson's "Behavioral Systems Model"
  6. M. Levine's "Conservation Theory"
  7. B. Neuman's "Health Care Systems Model"
  8. H. Peplau's "Interpersonal Relations in Nursing"
  9. J. Paterson's and L. Zderad's "Humanistic Nursing Theory"
  10. M. Leininger's "Culture Care Diversity and Universality"
  11. J. Watson's "Philosophy of Science and Caring"
  12. R. Parse's "Human Becoming Theory"
  13. M. Newman's "Health as Expanding Consciousness"
  14. A. Pender's "Health Promotion Model"

C. Examples of adapted frameworks
  1. A. Bandura's "Social Learning Theory"
  2. A. Maslow's "Hierarchy of Human Needs"
  3. L. Festinger's "Cognitive Dissonance"
  4. M. Seligman's "Helplessness"
  5. E. Duvall's and S. Minuchin's family theories
  6. V. Satir's "Family Communication Theory"
  7. R. Melzack's and D. Wall's "Pain"
  8. J. Piaget's, S. Freud's, and E. Erikson's developmental theories

---

CHECKLIST: CONCEPTUAL AND THEORETICAL FRAMEWORKS

Use the following questions to critique the conceptual or theoretical framework used in a study.

	Yes	No
• Is the framework clearly identified?	☐	☐
• Are the concepts and propositions clearly outlined?	☐	☐
• Does the framework appear to be appropriate for the research problem?	☐	☐
• Is sufficient literature presented to support and justify the framework?	☐	☐
• Did the researcher use a nursing framework or a borrowed framework?	☐	☐
• Does the link between the problem and the framework seem plausible and uncontrived?	☐	☐
• Does the hypothesis or research question flow naturally from the framework?	☐	☐
• Was the framework used to guide the research design, data collection and analysis, and interpretation of the findings?	☐	☐
• If the study findings do not support the framework, does the researcher suggest plausible explanations for this discrepancy?	☐	☐

---

    9. C. Spielberger's "Anxiety"
  10. I. Rosenstock's and M. Becker's "Health Beliefs and Compliance"
  11. R. Lazarus's and H. Selye's stress theories

V. Problems related to conceptual and theoretical frameworks

A. General information
    1. Framework problems typically result from researcher inexperience
    2. Such problems may limit the study's usefulness, because the findings may have no significance beyond the scope of the individual study
    3. Common problems include use of an inappropriate or unidentified framework in a study, use of a framework that is disconnected from the study, and use of multiple frameworks within the same study

B. Use of an inappropriate framework
    1. Typically occurs when the researcher tries to make a research problem fit within the context of a framework that may be only marginally related to the study
    2. Framework may be useless in interpreting the study's results

C. Use of a disconnected framework

1. Typically occurs when the researcher fails to connect an appropriately developed framework with the study
2. Framework has no meaning in the study and, consequently, is useless

D. Use of an unidentified framework
1. Typically occurs when the researcher fails to outline a framework
2. Results in findings that have no basis for generalizing to other situations

E. Use of multiple frameworks
1. Typically occurs when the researcher tries to use two or more frameworks for the same study
2. Framework has no meaning within the study because of the lack of logical connections between or among the frameworks (see *Checklist: Conceptual and Theoretical Frameworks*, page 37)

Points to remember

A framework gives direction to a study, provides a context for interpreting the findings, and adds to nursing's knowledge base.

Person, environment, health, and nursing — four key concepts of interest to nursing — are the focus of many frameworks used in research studies.

The main purpose of a conceptual or theoretical framework is to make research findings meaningful and generalizable.

A theoretical framework is more specific and concrete than a conceptual framework.

A model is a symbolic representation of a framework.

Use of an inappropriate or unidentified framework, a disconnected framework, or multiple frameworks within a study may compromise the study's usefulness.

Glossary

The following terms are defined in Appendix A, page 111.

concept	model
conceptual framework	proposition
hypothesis	theory

Study questions

To evaluate your understanding of this chapter, answer the following questions in the space provided; then compare your responses with the correct answers in Appendix B, page 116.

1. Which key concepts are of particular interest to nursing researchers? _____

   _____

   _____

2. What is the difference between a schematic model and a mathematical model? _____

   _____

   _____

3. What is the difference between the base for conceptual frameworks and the base for theoretical frameworks? _____

   _____

   _____

4. What are four nursing theories used to guide nursing research? _____

   _____

   _____

5. What are four theories borrowed from other disciplines used to guide nursing research? _____

   _____

   _____

6. What common problems are related to conceptual and theoretical frameworks? _____

   _____

   _____

CHAPTER 6

Variables, Hypotheses, and Research Questions

Learning objectives

Check off the following items once you've mastered them:

- [ ] Define *variable* and describe six types of variables used in hypotheses.

- [ ] Distinguish between the theoretical and operational definitions of variables.

- [ ] Discuss the purposes and sources of hypotheses.

- [ ] Identify the characteristics of a hypothesis.

- [ ] Distinguish among simple, complex, directional, nondirectional, research, and null hypotheses.

- [ ] Compare and contrast hypotheses and research questions.

- [ ] State the criteria for critiquing hypotheses and research questions.

I. Introduction

   A. QUANTITATIVE RESEARCH is based on the testability of relationships between the specific variables identified in a study

     1. A *variable* is a concept examined in a particular research study (for example, sex, age, heart rate, or pain perception)

     2. All variables must be concretely defined before they can be studied and measured

     3. Variables in qualitative studies may be abstract

   B. The researcher hypothesizes about the relationships between variables before beginning the study

     1. A *hypothesis* is a statement that predicts a relationship among two or more variables identified in the problem statement

     2. The hypothesis is more concise than the problem statement

   C. Research questions may be used instead of hypotheses whenever the researcher has insufficient knowledge to formulate a hypothesis; they are frequently used in qualitative research (see *Checklist: Hypotheses and Research Questions*)

II. Research variables

   A. General information

     1. All variables may be quantified and converted mathematically for statistical analysis

     2. All variables must be defined theoretically and operationally to reduce bias and clearly communicate meaning

     3. THEORETICAL DEFINITIONS, which are broad and abstract, derive from a specific theory or nursing-related literature; for example, "anxiety" may be defined theoretically as "a feeling of uneasiness or apprehension that affects body processes"

     4. OPERATIONAL DEFINITIONS reflect the procedures or acts that the researcher performs to measure the existence or degree of a variable; for example, "anxiety" may be defined operationally as "a state of mind that causes systolic blood pressure to increase at least 10 points"

   B. Types of variables

     1. An *independent* variable is the presumed cause manipulated by the researcher to observe the effect in a cause-and-effect relationship

     2. A *dependent* variable is the response or outcome the researcher wishes to explain or predict

     3. A *continuous* variable can take on a range of different values that can be represented on a continuum

     4. A *categorical* variable has a limited range of values that are represented by discrete categories

     5. An *extraneous* variable is a factor that can affect the dependent variable and interfere with the results

---

CHECKLIST: HYPOTHESES AND RESEARCH QUESTIONS

Use the following questions to critique the hypotheses and research questions found in a study.

	Yes	No
• Does the research report contain hypotheses or research questions?	☐	☐
• Do the hypotheses flow from the conceptual or theoretical framework or the literature review?	☐	☐
• Do the hypotheses predict solutions to the problem?	☐	☐
• Are the hypotheses clearly and objectively stated in a declarative form?	☐	☐
• Are the variables identified and potentially measurable?	☐	☐
• Do the hypotheses predict a relationship between the variables?	☐	☐
• Do the hypotheses indicate the population being studied?	☐	☐
• Are the hypotheses testable and clearly supported?	☐	☐
• If the hypotheses are nondirectional, did the researcher present a rationale to support their use?	☐	☐
• Are the hypotheses stated in the research form rather than the null form?	☐	☐
• Are the independent and dependent variables theoretically and operationally defined?	☐	☐
• Are the definitions consistent with the theoretical framework and the literature?	☐	☐

---

6. A *confounding* variable is an extraneous factor that has not been recognized or controlled

III. Hypotheses

A. General information

1. Hypotheses, formal statements of the expected relationships between the variables, provide direction for gathering and interpreting data; they are derived through inductive or deductive reasoning
2. The researcher should write the hypothesis before collecting the data and never alter the hypothesis after analyzing the data
3. The researcher should formulate as many hypotheses as needed to address all aspects of the research problem; the number of hypotheses formulated usually reflects the researcher's expertise and the complexity of the research problem

B. Purposes of hypotheses

    1. Help direct the research study by
      a. Identifying the population and specifying the variables
      b. Guiding the research design selection
      c. Suggesting an appropriate sampling technique and data collection
        and analysis methods
      d. Guiding the interpretation of results
    2. Help link theory to reality and, once confirmed, lend support to a
      theory

C. Sources of hypotheses
    1. Conceptual or theoretical frameworks, the most important sources,
      enable the researcher to derive hypotheses from concepts or theories
    2. Personal experience enables the researcher to induce hypotheses by
      observing events and explaining or predicting the relationship between
      events
    3. The literature review enables the researcher to formulate new
      hypotheses by regenerating hypotheses from other related studies or
      testing the assumptions underlying such studies

D. Characteristics of a hypothesis
    1. Written as a declarative sentence, commonly using a present-tense
      verb; content should be similar to that of the problem statement
    2. Identifies the population to be studied
    3. Identifies at least one independent variable and one dependent variable
    4. Is empirically testable and therefore cannot focus on moral or ethical
      issues

E. Types of hypotheses
    1. *Simple* hypothesis
      a. Easy to analyze
      b. Predicts a relationship between one independent variable and one
        dependent variable (for example, "a" is caused by "b")
    2. *Complex* hypothesis
      a. Predicts the relationships among two or more independent variables
        and two or more dependent variables (for example, "a" and "b" are
        caused by "c" and "d")
      b. Often used in nursing research because it typically examines
        complex human situations and requires the identification of several
        variables
    3. *Directional* hypothesis
      a. Can be simple or complex; predicts the direction of the relationship
        between the variables (for example, "a" is greater than "b")
      b. Form of most hypotheses deduced from theory
    4. *Nondirectional* hypothesis
      a. Can be simple or complex; states that a relationship exists between
        the variables (for example, "a" is related to "b")

      b. Typically used when not enough is known about the problem to predict the direction of a relationship
  5. *Research,* scientific, alternative, or theoretical hypothesis
      a. Can be simple or complex; usually is directional
      b. Anticipates a relationship between the variables
      c. Common form of hypotheses because of clarity
  6. *Null* or statistical hypothesis
      a. Predicts that no relationship exists between the independent and dependent variables
      b. Used whenever statistical principles are used to draw conclusions

IV. Research questions

A. General information
  1. The researcher may use a research question when knowledge is insufficient to formulate a hypothesis
  2. Research questions are commonly used in EXPLORATORY, DESCRIPTIVE, and QUALITATIVE RESEARCH
  3. Questions guiding qualitative research are usually broad and abstract

B. Characteristics of a research question
  1. Written as an interrogative sentence, using a present-tense verb
  2. Identifies the population
  3. Contains one or more variables
  4. Reflects the problem statement
  5. May or may not be empirically testable
  6. Focuses on the variables and their possible relationships

Points to remember

The researcher must be able to define the variables theoretically and operationally to test the hypothesis.

The hypothesis predicts relationships among two or more variables and identifies the population to be studied.

The hypothesis directs the research study and unifies theory and reality.

Hypotheses are never proven; they are accepted or rejected, or supported or not supported.

Hypotheses can be classified as simple, complex, directional, nondirectional, research, or null.

Research questions may be used in exploratory, descriptive, or qualitative research or when insufficient knowledge is available to formulate hypotheses.

Glossary

The following terms are defined in Appendix A, page 111.

descriptive research

exploratory research

operational definition

qualitative research

quantitative research

theoretical definition

Study questions

To evaluate your understanding of this chapter, answer the following questions in the space provided; then compare your responses with the correct answers in Appendix B, page 116.

1. What is the relationship between a variable and a hypothesis? _____

_____

_____

2. What is the difference between the theoretical and operational definitions of a variable? _____

_____

_____

3. What is the difference between the independent and the dependent variables?

_____

_____

4. Why would a researcher use a complex hypothesis? _____

_____

_____

5. How might research questions used to guide qualitative studies differ from those used in quantitative research? _____

_____

_____

CHAPTER 7

Research Designs

Learning objectives

Check off the following items once you've mastered them:

☐ Define *qualitative research* and *quantitative research*.

☐ Identify the threats to internal and external validity related to research design.

☐ Discuss each type of quantitative research design.

☐ Describe each type of qualitative research design.

☐ Compare and contrast qualitative and quantitative research designs.

☐ Compare and contrast cross-sectional and longitudinal designs and retrospective and prospective designs.

☐ Describe survey, methodological, case study, secondary analysis, and meta-analysis designs.

☐ State the criteria for critiquing quantitative, qualitative, and miscellaneous research designs.

I. Introduction

A. A research design is the logical plan used by the researcher to address the problem statement in a research study
   1. It follows an organized progression and takes the researcher from the research idea to the final step of the study
   2. It determines specific strategies for obtaining subjects, collecting data, analyzing data, and interpreting results

B. Choosing a research design is a major research decision

C. All research designs address six basic elements
   1. The setting in which the research occurs
   2. The subjects to include in the research
   3. The sample size or number of subjects in the study
   4. The conditions under which data are collected
   5. The methods used to collect the data
   6. The researcher's plan for analyzing the findings

D. Most research designs are categorized as either quantitative or qualitative
   1. *Quantitative* research, which is based on REDUCTIONISM, uses variables that are analyzed as numbers
   2. *Qualitative* research, which is based on HOLISM, uses concepts that are analyzed as words to identify the relationships among variables
   3. Many researchers think that qualitative research is more consistent with nursing's philosophical basis; others think that quantitative research is more rigorous and scientific
   4. Quantitative research designs usually are best suited to studies that focus on determining causes and effects; qualitative research designs, to studies that focus on discovery or exploration
   5. Some researchers advocate integrating quantitative and qualitative research within a study or group of studies to enhance the knowledge gained

E. The researcher may also use triangulation
   1. *Triangulation* is a strategy in which multiple methods are used in the research design to study the phenomenon and converge on the truth
   2. There are five types of triangulation
      a. In data triangulation, data from several sources in a study are examined
      b. In investigator triangulation, several investigators with differing backgrounds examine the same variables
      c. In theoretical triangulation, several frameworks or perspectives are used in a study
      d. In methodological triangulation, several methods, such as observations, interviews, and questionnaires, are used to collect data from the same subjects in a study

    e. In analysis triangulation, different techniques are used to analyze the same data

II. Quantitative research designs

A. General information
1. The quantitative research design evolves from the hypothesis and determines which methods and procedures will be used to select subjects, collect and analyze data, and interpret results
2. The main purposes are to help the researcher find a solution to the research problem and maintain control over all variables
3. Quantitative designs differ according to the degree of control the researcher has over the variables; the degree of control directly affects the internal and external validity of the study—two areas that help to determine whether the study results are credible and dependable
   a. *Internal validity*, the extent to which the effects detected in the study are a reflection of reality, depends on whether the independent variable affects the dependent variable in some way
   b. *External validity*, the extent to which the findings can be generalized beyond the sample used in the study, depends on whether the relationship between the independent and dependent variables can be applied to other populations or situations
   c. Factors other than the independent variable that affect the study results are referred to as *threats*
      (1) Threats to internal validity
         (a) History
         (b) Maturation
         (c) Testing
         (d) Instrumentation
         (e) Mortality or attrition
         (f) Selection bias
      (2) Threats to external validity
         (a) Sample inadequacy
         (b) Environmental influence
4. Techniques used to control threats include the following
   a. *Randomization* is the random assignment of subjects to a group, with each individual in the population having an equal chance to be selected for the group
   b. *Homogeneity* is the selection for participation in a study of only those subjects who share an extraneous variable—for example, only men or only adults over age 65
   c. *Blocking* is the purposeful addition of an extraneous variable to the study's design—for example, random assignment of men and women to separate groups

  d. *Matching* is the formation of a comparison group by matching
     subjects on the basis of important extraneous variables—for
     example, age, sex, and health status
  e. *Analysis of covariance* is the control of extraneous variables
     through statistical procedures
5. Quantitative research designs can be classified as true experimental,
   quasi-experimental, pre-experimental, and nonexperimental

B. True experimental designs
  1. A *true experimental design*, which offers the greatest amount of
     control and minimal threat to internal validity, allows the researcher
     to become actively involved in the study
  2. Characteristics of a true experimental design include the following
     a. *Manipulation*—the researcher manipulates the independent variable
        so that some of the subjects are affected
     b. *Control*—the researcher uses one or more measures to control the
        experiment, including the use of an unmanipulated control group
        that is compared with an experimental group
     c. *Randomization*—the researcher assigns subjects to groups by
        chance
  3. True experimental designs are the most effective method of testing
     cause-and-effect relationships
  4. *Causality* is based on meeting three criteria
     a. The cause must precede the effect
     b. An empirical relationship between the presumed cause and effect
        must exist
     c. The relationship cannot be attributable to the effect of a third
        variable
  5. True experimental designs can be classified into three types
     a. In a *pretest–post-test control group design*, the researcher randomly
        assigns each subject to either a control group or an experimental
        group
        (1) Both groups are given a pretest, after which only the
            experimental group receives a specific intervention that is
            manipulated by the researcher
        (2) Both groups are then given a post-test
        (3) The researcher examines the performances of both groups for
            changes in scores that may have resulted from the intervention
     b. In a *post-test–only control group design*, the researcher randomly
        assigns each subject to either a control group or an experimental
        group
        (1) After the experimental group receives a specific intervention,
            both groups are given a post-test
        (2) The researcher then examines the performances of both
            groups for differences in scores that may have resulted from
            the intervention

    c. In a *Solomon four-group design,* the researcher randomly assigns each subject to one of two control groups or one of two experimental groups
       (1) Only one control group or one experimental group is given the pretest, and both experimental groups receive a specific intervention
       (2) All groups are given a post-test
       (3) The researcher examines the performances of all the groups for the effect of the pretest on post-test scores and for any other differences among the groups
  6. Use of true experimental designs is limiting for a number of reasons
    a. Certain variables (such as age, sex, and height) cannot be physically manipulated
    b. Other variables (such as disease or unhealthy habits) cannot be ethically manipulated
    c. True experimentation may be impossible in particular settings
    d. The HAWTHORNE EFFECT may interfere with the study's outcome
    e. Some researchers consider true experiments artificial and reductionistic

C. Quasi-experimental designs
  1. A *quasi-experimental design* is used to test cause-and-effect relationships when true experimentation is impossible
    a. It is more conducive to a natural setting
    b. It allows the researcher to become actively involved in the study and to generalize the findings to an extent
  2. Unlike a true experimental design, a quasi-experimental design does not depend on randomization or control; however, it does allow for manipulation of the independent variable and enables the researcher to introduce other factors to compensate for the lack of randomization or a control group
  3. Typically, the researcher uses a comparison group instead of a control group to evaluate outcome differences
  4. Quasi-experimental designs can be classified into two types
    a. A *nonequivalent control group design* is identical to the pretest–post-test control group of a true experimental design except that the subjects are not randomly assigned to groups
       (1) The researcher cannot assume that both groups are equal
       (2) The researcher therefore must rely on the results of a pretest to determine if groups are initially similar with respect to the dependent variable
    b. A *time series design* involves the collection of information from one group of subjects at several points over an extended period

      (1) The researcher introduces an intervention at a specific time during the course of data collection and evaluates the results based on information collected before and after the intervention

      (2) Although subjects are not randomly assigned, this design allows the researcher to manipulate factors to control the study

  5. Use of quasi-experimental designs is limiting for two reasons

    a. The researcher cannot draw inferences about cause-and-effect relationships to the same degree as in true experimental designs

    b. The researcher has limited control over variables, which may necessitate formulating alternative explanations for the effect detected in the study

D. Pre-experimental designs

  1. A *pre-experimental design,* which may be used when a control group is impossible or when limited opportunities for data collection are available, is typically more economical than a true experimental design or a quasi-experimental design

  2. Pre-experimental designs can be classified according to two types: post-test–only nonequivalent control group and one-group pretest–post-test

    a. A *post-test–only nonequivalent control group design* is similar to a nonequivalent control group design except that the researcher has no pre-test data with which to compare the groups' relationship to the dependent variable and has no basis on which to judge the initial equivalence or similarity of the two groups involved in the study

    b. A *one-group pretest–post-test design* does not depend on the use of randomization or a comparison group; after the group is given a pretest, the researcher introduces an intervention and then administers a post-test to examine changes between pretest and post-test scores

  3. Use of pre-experimental designs is limiting because the researcher cannot determine cause-and-effect relationships and may be unable to rule out alternative explanations for the effect detected in the study

E. Nonexperimental designs

  1. In a *nonexperimental design,* the researcher collects data without making changes or introducing an intervention

    a. It is an efficient and effective way of collecting a large amount of information about a problem in a realistic setting

    b. This type of design allows the researcher to investigate complex relationships among variables and to develop a foundation for future experimental studies

---

CHECKLIST: QUANTITATIVE RESEARCH DESIGNS

Use the following questions to critique the quantitative research design used in a study.

General questions	Yes	No
• Is the most appropriate design used for the research problem?	☐	☐
• Does the design flow from the problem statement, literature review, theoretical framework, and hypothesis?	☐	☐
• Is the design realistic?	☐	☐
• Does the researcher use control methods to enhance internal and external validity?	☐	☐
• If a stronger design could have been used, does the researcher justify use of the weaker design?	☐	☐
• Are the major limitations of the selected design considered when interpreting the results?	☐	☐

True experimental design

	Yes	No
• Was a true experimental design used?	☐	☐
• Does the design address a cause-and-effect relationship?	☐	☐
• Is the researcher's use of manipulation, control, and randomization clear?	☐	☐
• Is the intervention described in detail?	☐	☐
• Are any alternative explanations for the results presented?	☐	☐
• Are the findings generalizable to the larger population?	☐	☐

Quasi-experimental and pre-experimental designs

	Yes	No
• Was a quasi-experimental or pre-experimental design used?	☐	☐
• Could the researcher have used a true experimental design instead?	☐	☐
• Were the most common threats to the internal and external validity of the study identified?	☐	☐
• Have all possible alternative explanations been satisfactorily discounted?	☐	☐
• Is the intervention described in detail?	☐	☐

(continued)

2. The researcher may use this type of design when the independent variable cannot be manipulated or should not be manipulated because of ethical considerations or when use of a true experimental or quasi-experimental design is impractical, undesirable, or inappropriate

---

CHECKLIST: QUANTITATIVE RESEARCH DESIGNS *(continued)*

Nonexperimental design	Yes	No
• Was a nonexperimental design used?	☐	☐
• Is the design appropriate for the study?	☐	☐
• Does the researcher discuss the findings in a manner congruous with the design?	☐	☐
• Does the researcher attempt to infer cause-and-effect relationships?	☐	☐
• Does the researcher discuss threats to internal and external validity?	☐	☐
• Are alternative explanations addressed?	☐	☐

---

3. Nonexperimental designs can be classified according to three types: correlational, ex post facto, and descriptive
    a. A *correlational design* is typically used to examine the relationship between two variables to see if, when one variable changes, the other variable also changes
    b. An *ex post facto design* is typically used to investigate the effect on the dependent variable of a change in the independent variable; the researcher may use comparison groups in this type of design
    c. A *descriptive design* is typically used to observe, describe, or document aspects of a situation; this type of design does not concern the relationship between variables
    d. Use of nonexperimental designs is limiting for two reasons
        (1) The researcher cannot establish cause-and-effect relationships or determine why the variables respond as they do
        (2) The researcher also may be unable to rule out alternative explanations for the effects detected in the study and may have difficulty interpreting the findings (see *Checklist: Quantitative Research Designs*)

III. Qualitative research designs

A. General information
    1. Qualitative research designs, relatively new to nursing research, provide insight, meaning, and understanding about a subject's experiences
    2. The researcher typically conducts a literature review after the data collection and analysis to avoid being influenced by preconceived expectations

3. Intuition and empathy play key roles in qualitative research; the researcher typically becomes closely involved with the subjects in an attempt to understand their thoughts and ideas and must develop and cultivate intuitive and empathic feelings to prompt further dialogue
4. Qualitative research designs have five primary purposes
   a. Describing phenomena
   b. Generating hypotheses
   c. Illustrating the meanings of relationships
   d. Understanding relationships
   e. Developing, refining, or expanding theory
5. Concepts important to qualitative research designs include gestalt, bracketing, and intuiting
   a. *Gestalt* refers to the clustering of knowledge about a particular phenomenon into linked ideas to enhance meaning; qualitative research forms new gestalts to generate new theories
   b. *Bracketing* refers to the putting aside of what is known about a phenomenon to allow the researcher to observe it without preconceptions and to form new gestalts
   c. *Intuiting* refers to the process of examining the phenomenon being studied; this requires the researcher's concentration and complete absorption to focus on the area of interest
6. Qualitative research designs can be classified into six major categories: phenomenological, grounded theory, ethnographic, historical, philosophical inquiry, and critical social theory

B. Phenomenological research design
   1. *Phenomenological research* is based on the belief that no single reality exists and that individuals have separate and unique realities
   2. This design can enhance understanding through real-life experiences as described by participating subjects or informants; the researcher attempts to derive meaning by perceiving through the subject's reality
   3. The researcher identifies the phenomenon or experience to be explored and formulates one or more research questions; subjects are chosen based on their willingness to share personal experiences and feelings
   4. The researcher may use a combination of strategies to collect the data; data collection and analysis may occur simultaneously (see Chapters 9 and 10 for further details on data collection and analysis)
   5. Throughout the study, the researcher focuses on the actual experience, including which aspects of the experience the subjects perceive to be important and which changes or outcomes result from the experience
   6. Study findings may be described from the subjects' viewpoints
   7. Important considerations include maintaining a relaxed environment to elicit feelings about an experience and using bracketing and intuiting throughout the study

C. Grounded theory research design
   1. *Grounded theory research* is used to generate new theory from data collected without the aid of a pre-existing theory as a framework
   2. The researcher, who uses a combination of inductive and deductive reasoning, must remain open-minded about the findings
   3. This type of design is most useful in studying areas that have not been previously researched or in gaining a new viewpoint in known areas
   4. Intuiting plays an important role in grounded theory research
   5. Unlike the systematically arranged steps of other types of research, the steps in grounded theory research occur simultaneously; the researcher typically observes situations, collects data, organizes the data, and analyzes the data all at the same time
   6. The researcher collects data through observations, interviews, or examination of pre-existing records and frequently relies on handwritten notes and tape recordings as a means of recording the data
   7. The researcher attempts to collect data from as many diverse sources as possible to understand the situation fully; amassed data may be voluminous
   8. The researcher analyzes the data using the constant comparative method (see Chapter 10 for further information)

D. Ethnographic research design
   1. *Ethnographic research* evolved from anthropology and involves the study of individuals or artifacts in a natural or real setting
   2. Ethnographic research is primarily used to describe culture and is particularly helpful in the study of specific life-styles or cultural phenomena from the subjects' viewpoints
   3. In this type of research, the researcher becomes totally involved in the setting during data collection in an attempt to understand the daily life of the individual or group being studied but must maintain objectivity to avoid being assimilated into the culture or group
   4. At the beginning of an ethnographic study, the researcher identifies the culture or group to be studied as well as any significant variables within the culture or group, then conducts a literature review to learn as much as possible about what is already known about the culture or group
   5. After gaining access to the culture or group, the researcher becomes immersed in the culture and tries to gain the confidence and support of individuals who are willing to explain cultural phenomena
   6. Because extensive note taking is required during data collection, the researcher relies on intuition to determine which data to gather
   7. The researcher typically uses direct observation to gather data; a description of the culture or group usually evolves from the data
   8. The researcher develops theories to explain the relationships revealed by the data, which may lead to the formation of new hypotheses

E. Historical research design
   1. *Historical research*, the careful examination and analysis of data from the past, is used to provide an understanding of the effect of the past on present and future events
   2. This type of design is primarily based on the study of written materials; however, oral reports, photographs, films, and other artifacts also serve as sources of information
   3. At the beginning of a historical study, the researcher formulates an idea, then clearly defines and narrows it to ensure that a search for related materials is realistic; afterward, the researcher develops general research questions to guide the study
   4. After conducting a literature review, the researcher identifies and locates available sources, such as in private archives or libraries
   5. After collecting the data, the researcher evaluates the information using external and internal criticism
      a. *External criticism* determines the data's genuineness and authenticity (validity)
      b. *Internal criticism* determines the data's truth and accuracy (reliability)
   6. Collection of data may take months or years and may not have an obvious end
   7. In analyzing the data, the researcher must clarify any conflicting evidence and decide which data to accept or reject as part of the findings
   8. The written research report may be in the form of a biography or chronology, or it may focus on a particular issue

F. Philosophical inquiry research design
   1. *Philosophical inquiry research* is conducted to debate issues or develop theories; analysis is used to examine the nature of values, ethics, and knowledge
   2. The researcher uses inquiry and analysis to examine an issue from all perspectives
   3. Philosophical questions guide the research, with data collection and analysis occurring simultaneously; answers generate additional questions that result in further analysis, creating a cyclical process
   4. The researcher often discusses the analysis of questions and answers with colleagues
   5. Reports focus on the conclusions of the analysis rather than on the methodology used
   6. There are three types of philosophical inquiry
      a. Foundational inquiry examines the foundations of a science
      b. Philosophical analysis examines meanings
      c. Ethical analysis examines morality

G. Critical social theory research design

CHECKLIST: QUALITATIVE RESEARCH DESIGNS

Use the following questions to critique the qualitative research design used in a study.

General questions	**Yes**	**No**
• Does the research question seem to explore, describe, or expand knowledge about the phenomenon of interest?	☐	☐
• Is the most appropriate design used for the study?	☐	☐
• Has the research question been previously researched?	☐	☐
• Is the research question congruous with the philosophical basis of holism?	☐	☐
• Does evidence suggest that the researcher used bracketing and intuiting to form new gestalts about the phenomenon?	☐	☐

Phenomenological research design		
• Does the study examine the phenomenon from the subject's or informant's perspective?	☐	☐
• Is the researcher an active participant in the subject's world?	☐	☐
• Has the researcher attempted to seek out individuals who are willing to share their feelings about the experience?	☐	☐
• Were the data collection methods appropriate?	☐	☐
• Did data collection and analysis occur simultaneously?	☐	☐
• Were the results described from the subjects or informant's viewpoint?	☐	☐

Grounded theory research design		
• Is the study phenomenon clearly identified?	☐	☐
• Has the phenomenon been previously researched?	☐	☐
• Is the researcher offering a fresh viewpoint or a familiar topic of interest?	☐	☐
• Does the researcher attempt to develop a theory about the phenomenon?	☐	☐
• Are data collection and recording methods appropriate for the situation?	☐	☐
• Does evidence suggest that the data were collected from as many sources as possible?	☐	☐
• Has the researcher collected, organized, and analyzed the data simultaneously?	☐	☐

(continued)

CHECKLIST: QUALITATIVE RESEARCH DESIGNS *(continued)*

	Yes	No
Ethnographic research design		
• Is the study conducted in a natural setting?	☐	☐
• Is the researcher totally involved in the setting during data collection?	☐	☐
• Does the researcher attempt to understand the subject's or informant's view and to describe the culture?	☐	☐
• Did the researcher become part of the culture?	☐	☐
• Did the researcher maintain objectivity?	☐	☐
• Did the researcher obtain the support and confidence of the subjects?	☐	☐
• Were data collection methods appropriate for the situation?	☐	☐
Historical research design		
• Does the study attempt to provide an understanding of how the past has influenced present or possible future events?	☐	☐
• Has the researcher clearly defined and narrowed the topic being studied?	☐	☐
• Were historical materials adequately analyzed and all possible sources of data explored?	☐	☐
• Has the researcher subjected the data to external and internal criticism?	☐	☐
• Did the researcher reconcile conflicting data and provide a valid rationale for drawing conclusions based on the study's findings?	☐	☐
Philosophical inquiry research design		
• Does the research debate an issue or examine the nature of values, ethics, or knowledge?	☐	☐
• Has the researcher analyzed the issue from all perspectives?	☐	☐
• Did the researcher use philosophical questions to guide the study?	☐	☐
• Did data collection and analysis occur simultaneously?	☐	☐
• Did the researcher focus on the conclusions of the analysis?	☐	☐
Critical social theory research design		
• Does the research explore a facet of society in which there are patterns of domination?	☐	☐
• Has the researcher exposed constraints that impede free and equal participation in society?	☐	☐
• Does the researcher seek to facilitate liberation and authenticity?	☐	☐

1. *Critical social theory research* is based on the belief that most societies function within patterns of domination and inhibit personal growth of individuals; certain societal facts are taken for granted and are not questioned or disputed
2. The researcher tries to understand how people develop symbolic meanings and to expose the constraints that impede free and equal participation in society
3. Using the structures of society, the researcher exposes issues of privilege, exploitation, and oppression to facilitate liberation and authenticity
4. Social structures of interest to nurses include images of women, health care delivery, families, and minorities
5. Feminist research uses critical social theory methods (see *Checklist: Qualitative Research Designs*)

IV. Other research designs

A. General information
   1. Other research designs may be used with quantitative or qualitative designs to provide the researcher with additional guidance
   2. Other commonly used research designs include cross-sectional, longitudinal, retrospective, prospective, survey, methodological, case study, secondary analysis, and meta-analysis

B. Cross-sectional research designs
   1. A *cross-sectional research design* involves the simultaneous collection of data from different subjects at different stages of the same phenomenon to provide a total representation of the phenomenon
   2. This type of design is typically used in conjunction with a nonexperimental research design
   3. A cross-sectional design has three major advantages
      a. The design is practical and relatively manageable
      b. The researcher can use time efficiently and collect voluminous data economically
      c. Maturation is eliminated as a threat to internal validity
   4. A cross-sectional design also has three limitations
      a. The design structure may imply that differences between groups of subjects are attributable to time rather than generational variances
      b. Several alternative explanations may account for the observed differences
      c. The researcher cannot perform a detailed analysis of the interrelationships among the phenomena being studied

C. Longitudinal research designs
   1. A *longitudinal research design* involves the collection of data from the same subjects over time to provide information on changes or trends

2. This type of design is typically used in conjunction with a nonexperimental design
3. Longitudinal designs can be classified into three types: panel studies, trend studies, and follow-up studies
    a. In a *panel study*, the researcher collects data from the same sample of subjects at two or more times
    b. In a *trend study*, the researcher collects data from different samples of subjects from the same population at two or more times
    c. In a *follow-up study*, the researcher collects data from the same sample of subjects, usually at a later time
4. A longitudinal design has four major advantages
    a. The design is useful in studying the interrelationships among variables over time
    b. The researcher can more accurately study changes that occur over time
    c. The timing of phenomena can be more easily determined
    d. The subjects can serve as their own controls
5. A longitudinal design also has three major limitations
    a. Loss of subjects (mortality) is a common threat to internal validity
    b. Data collection may be expensive and time-consuming
    c. Several alternative explanations may account for observed differences

D. Retrospective research designs
1. A *retrospective research design* involves the collection of data about subjects' pasts (antecedent factors) to determine which factors, if any, precipitated or contributed to a current phenomenon
2. This type of design, basically epidemiologic in nature, is typically used in conjunction with a nonexperimental (specifically, ex post facto) research design
3. A retrospective design makes the researcher's work easier and more efficient in three areas
    a. The collection of voluminous data
    b. The exploration of complex relationships
    c. The generation of hypotheses that might provide a foundation for future experimental studies
4. A retrospective design also has three major limitations
    a. The researcher cannot establish direct cause-and-effect relationships
    b. Many alternative explanations for results cannot be ruled out
    c. Findings may be difficult to interpret because the variables may be interrelated in complex ways

E. Prospective research designs
1. A *prospective research design* involves tracking subjects to observe for a phenomenon whose presumed cause has been identified
2. The purpose of a prospective design is to attempt to establish a stronger case for a cause-and-effect relationship

3. This type of design, basically epidemiologic in nature, may be used in conjunction with experimental, quasi-experimental, or nonexperimental research designs
4. A prospective design has three major advantages
   a. Questions involving the timing of events are easily resolved, because the independent variable can be manipulated to later observe for the dependent variable
   b. There is an increased likelihood that samples are representative of the population
   c. The researcher can impose controls that help rule out alternative explanations for the observed effects
5. A prospective design also has four major limitations
   a. The design is typically costly and time-consuming
   b. Loss of subjects is a threat to internal validity
   c. Alternative explanations for the observed results are possible if the research is quasi-experimental or nonexperimental
   d. A large sample of subjects is needed to conduct the study
F. Survey research designs
   1. A *survey research design* involves data collection from a sample of subjects to examine the opinions, attitudes, behaviors, or characteristics of the population
   2. A survey is similar to a *census* except that in a census, the researcher collects data from each member of the population
   3. Data collection methods used in survey research include face-to-face interviews, telephone interviews, and written questionnaires
      a. *Face-to-face interviews* are the most effective means of conducting a survey because of the quality and amount of information obtained; however, they require much planning, interview training, and time
      b. *Telephone interviews* are typically an easy approach to collecting much information rapidly; however, subjects may be uncooperative and unresponsive
      c. *Questionnaires* are self-administered surveys that provide clear, simple, and unambiguous answers about subject characteristics; although economical and easily distributed through the mail, questionnaires may have a low return rate
   4. A survey design has three major advantages
      a. The researcher can easily obtain voluminous data from many subjects
      b. The researcher can reach many populations and cover a wide range of topics
      c. The design's methodology can be easily stated so that the research is easier to evaluate and replicate
   5. A survey design also has five major limitations
      a. Subjects may be reluctant to share certain information about themselves

      b. The information obtained tends to be superficial

      c. The researcher cannot draw cause-and-effect conclusions

      d. The survey may require much time and money

      e. Especially with questionnaires, a low response rate is possible

G. Methodological research designs

    1. A *methodological research design* involves the development, testing, and evaluation of research instruments to develop reliable and valid research tools and techniques

    2. This type of design, which is primarily concerned with the means by which researchers collect, organize, and analyze data, may be used with experimental, quasi-experimental, or nonexperimental designs

    3. The researcher using a methodological design must be knowledgeable about PSYCHOMETRIC PROPERTIES

    4. Methodological studies are particularly important in new fields, such as nursing research, that focus on complex, intangible phenomena

    5. A methodological design has three major advantages

      a. The researcher can provide reliable and valid instruments greatly needed by other nursing researchers

      b. Newly discovered or invented instruments are immediately applicable

      c. The study can provide direction for other substantive research

    6. A methodological design also has two major limitations

      a. Such studies are typically time-consuming and may become a researcher's lifework

      b. The new instrument may require many revisions with subsequent testing before it can be used by other researchers

H. Case study research designs

    1. A *case study research design* involves the detailed investigation of an individual, group, or institution to understand which variables are important to the subject's history, development, or care

    2. The researcher typically focuses on understanding why the subject thinks, behaves, or develops in a particular manner

    3. A case study design has two major advantages

      a. The researcher may obtain detailed information about the subject, insight into complex relationships, and direction for future research

      b. The study can be conducted over time

    4. A case study design also has three major limitations

      a. The researcher's familiarity with the subject makes objectivity difficult

      b. The results lack generalizability

      c. Cause-and-effect relationships cannot be determined

I. Secondary analysis research designs

    1. A *secondary analysis research design* involves further examination of previously collected data

CHECKLIST: MISCELLANEOUS RESEARCH DESIGNS

Use the following questions to critique a miscellaneous research design in a study.

	Yes	No
Cross-sectional research design		
• Does the use of a cross-sectional approach seem appropriate?	☐	☐
• Were the data collected from all subjects at one time?	☐	☐
• Is a nonexperimental design used?	☐	☐
• Does the researcher identify alternative explanations for the results?	☐	☐
Longitudinal research design		
• Does the use of a longitudinal research design seem appropriate?	☐	☐
• Do the number of data collection points and the time intervals between data collections seem appropriate for the study?	☐	☐
• Was a panel, trend, or follow-up study used?	☐	☐
• Is a nonexperimental design used?	☐	☐
• Does the researcher identify alternative explanations for the results?	☐	☐
• Does the researcher address the problem of subject loss (mortality)?	☐	☐
Retrospective research design		
• Does the use of a retrospective research design seem appropriate?	☐	☐
• Has the researcher attempted to determine which past factors might have precipitated the present phenomenon?	☐	☐
• Does the study use an epidemiological or a nonexperimental design?	☐	☐
• Does the researcher suggest hypotheses that could be tested in future research studies?	☐	☐
• Does the researcher identify alternative explanations for the results?	☐	☐
Prospective research design		
• Does a prospective research design seem appropriate for the study?	☐	☐
• Are selected subjects followed over time and observed for the occurrence of the phenomenon of interest?	☐	☐
• Does the researcher impose controls to rule out alternative explanations for the results obtained?	☐	☐
• Does the study use an experimental, a quasi-experimental, or a nonexperimental design?	☐	☐

(continued)

CHECKLIST: MISCELLANEOUS RESEARCH DESIGNS *(continued)*

	Yes	No
Survey research design		
• Does the study lend itself to a survey?	☐	☐
• Was an appropriate data collection approach used?	☐	☐
• Was it the best one for the problem?	☐	☐
• Does the researcher clearly describe the contents of the survey and the methodology used?	☐	☐
• Does the researcher try to infer cause-and-effect relationships?	☐	☐
• Is the response rate specified?	☐	☐
• Does the researcher offer alternative explanations for the findings?	☐	☐
Methodological research design		
• Is the development of a reliable and valid instrument the focus?	☐	☐
• Does the study identify and define the concept to be measured?	☐	☐
• Are the results of reliability and validity tests reported?	☐	☐
Case study research design		
• Does the research involve a detailed investigation of an individual, a group, or an institution?	☐	☐
• Are the data collection methods clearly described and appropriate?	☐	☐
• Has the researcher avoided bias in presenting the findings?	☐	☐
• Does the researcher overgeneralize the findings?	☐	☐
Secondary analysis research design		
• Does the researcher identify the source of data used for the secondary analysis?	☐	☐
• Is the purpose of the analysis specified?	☐	☐
• Does a secondary analysis seem appropriate for the study?	☐	☐
Meta-analysis research design		
• Does the researcher integrate findings from several research studies?	☐	☐
• Has the researcher attempted to obtain all research (published and unpublished) related to the variables of interest?	☐	☐
• Is the effect size for each study calculated?	☐	☐
• Does the researcher describe the study's limitations?	☐	☐
• Does the researcher overgeneralize the findings?	☐	☐

2. Variables not analyzed in an original research study are prime targets for a secondary analysis
3. A secondary analysis design can be a powerful research tool if the researcher uses two or more sets of data with comparable variables
4. A secondary analysis design has three major advantages
    a. The research can be efficiently and economically conducted
    b. The researcher can bypass the data collection phase
    c. Data are not wasted
5. A secondary analysis design also has three major limitations
    a. The data may not contain all the information desired for analysis
    b. The researcher runs the risk of using inaccurate data
    c. Data relevant to the research topic may be difficult or impossible to find
J. Meta-analysis research designs
    1. A *meta-analysis research design* involves the merging of findings from several studies that have examined the same variables to integrate the findings and enhance their total contribution
    2. In a meta-analysis study, the researcher calculates a statistic (EFFECT SIZE) for the dependent variable of each study
    3. A meta-analysis design has three major advantages
        a. The researcher can integrate voluminous data objectively
        b. The researcher may discover new patterns and relationships that might otherwise have gone unnoticed
        c. Information obtained may be used in theory and future research development
    4. A meta-analysis design also has three major limitations
        a. Studies may be combined that conceptually do not belong together
        b. The results may be biased toward studies with only significant findings, because unpublished data probably will not be included
        c. A research report may not contain sufficient information for the researcher to compute an effect size (See *Checklist: Miscellaneous Research Designs*)

Points to remember

The research design is the researcher's overall plan for obtaining answers to the research problem; choosing a research design is a major research decision.

Qualitative research designs are based on holism, which focuses on the study of the total experience; quantitative research designs are based on reductionism, which focuses on the study of parts.

Common threats to internal validity include history, maturation, testing, instrumentation, mortality, and selection bias.

Common threats to external validity include adequacy of the population sample and environmental characteristics.

True experimental research designs offer the greatest control over variables.

Cross-sectional research designs collect data at one time; longitudinal research designs collect data several times.

Retrospective research designs attempt to identify factors in a subject's past that might have precipitated a current phenomenon; prospective research follows a subject over time to observe for an effect whose presumed cause has been identified.

Glossary

The following terms are defined in Appendix A, page 111.

effect size

Hawthorne effect

holism

psychometric properties

reductionism

Study questions

To evaluate your understanding of this chapter, answer the following questions in the space provided; then compare your responses with the correct answers in Appendix B, pages 116 and 117.

1. What is the difference between quantitative and qualitative research?

_____

_____

2. What are six threats to internal validity? _____

_____

_____

3. What are the characteristics of a true experimental design? _____

_____

_____

4. What are six major categories of a qualitative research design? _____

_____

_____

5. What is the difference between cross-sectional and longitudinal research designs? _____

_____

6. Which data collection methods are used in survey research designs? _____

_____

_____

7. Which research design involves the development, testing, and evaluation of research instruments? _____

_____

CHAPTER 8

Sampling Techniques

Learning objectives

Check off the following items once you've mastered them:

☐ Define *population*.

☐ Identify the factors to consider when selecting a sample.

☐ Outline the steps used in selecting a sample.

☐ Discuss the four types of probability sampling techniques: simple random, stratified random, cluster, and systematic.

☐ Describe the four types of nonprobability sampling techniques: accidental, quota, purposive, and network.

☐ Compare and contrast probability and nonprobability sampling techniques.

☐ State the criteria for critiquing sampling techniques.

I. Introduction

A. The following terms are commonly used in sampling
1. *Population* — entire group of ELEMENTS that meets a well-defined set of eligibility criteria; a population may consist of people, animals, objects, words, or events
2. *Eligibility criteria* — descriptors chosen by the researcher to define which elements should be included in or excluded from the population
3. *Sampling* — process of selecting a portion of the population to represent the entire population
4. *Sample* — subset of elements from the population
5. *Representative sample* — group of elements whose characteristics closely match those of the population
6. *Stratum* — mutually exclusive segment of the population (subpopulation) based on one or more characteristics, such as race or sex; strata are used to improve the representativeness of a sample
7. *Bias* — overrepresentation or underrepresentation of some segment or characteristic of a population in a research study
8. *Sampling frame* — list of all the elements in the population
9. *Sampling error* — difference between population values and sample values; the larger the sampling error, the less representative the sample is of the population

B. Sampling is used by researchers because it is an economical and efficient means of collecting data and because collecting data from the entire population usually is not necessary or feasible

C. The sampling technique, integral to the research, may affect the study's outcome
1. The criteria used to define the population affect the generalizability of the findings
2. The use of a sample that exhibits HOMOGENEITY with respect to key variables may result in researcher bias, a potential threat to the study's validity
3. The use of a sample that does not reflect the same variations as that of the population may lead to inconclusive findings

D. The researcher typically determines the sample size before collecting data

E. The researcher should consider several factors when selecting a sample: the type of sampling; the HETEROGENEITY of the variables being investigated; frequency of occurrence of the variable of interest; and the cost

F. Using the largest sample possible is usually best
1. Generally, the larger the sample, the more representative it will be
2. At least 10, but preferably 20 to 30, subjects should be selected for every variable or subset of data
3. The researcher may be able to estimate the sample size needed using a statistical procedure known as POWER ANALYSIS

CHECKLIST: SAMPLING TECHNIQUES

Use the following questions to critique the sampling technique used in a study.

	Yes	No
• Is the population identified?	☐	☐
• Are the eligibility criteria specified?	☐	☐
• Are the sample selection techniques adequately described so that the sampling procedure can be replicated?	☐	☐
• Is a probability or nonprobability sampling technique used?	☐	☐
• Is the sample representative of the population?	☐	☐
• If any biases were introduced by the sampling technique, has the researcher identified them?	☐	☐
• Are the characteristics and size of the sample described?	☐	☐
• Is the sample size sufficient?	☐	☐
• Can the results be generalized to the population from which the sample was drawn?	☐	☐

   G. Seven steps are involved in sampling
      1. Identifying and defining the population
      2. Delineating the accessible portion of the population
      3. Deciding how to choose the sample
      4. Determining the sample size, using power analysis if possible
      5. Obtaining permission from the human subjects committee or institutional review board to conduct the study
      6. Recruiting the subjects and obtaining informed consent
      7. Estimating the representativeness of the sample

   H. The two basic sampling techniques used in nursing research are probability (RANDOM) sampling and nonprobability (nonrandom) sampling (see *Checklist: Sampling Techniques*)

II. Probability (random) sampling

   A. General information
      1. Probability sampling involves the selection of elements from the population using random procedures in which each element of the population has an equal and independent chance of being chosen
      2. Probability sampling is the only method of obtaining a representative sample, because the use of random techniques eliminates the possibility of researcher bias on a conscious and an unconscious level

3. When using probability sampling, the researcher can estimate the degree of sampling error
4. Probability sampling is important to the use of most statistical tests
5. Probability sampling, although preferred, has drawbacks
    a. It is expensive and inconvenient
    b. It may be impractical or unnecessary for certain studies
    c. The researcher has no guarantee that all randomly chosen subjects will participate in the study
6. Probability sampling can be further classified into four types: simple random, stratified random, cluster (multi-stage), and systematic

B. Simple random sampling
    1. *Simple random sampling* allows the researcher to select elements randomly from a sampling frame
    2. Typically, the researcher lists all of the elements of the population, numbers the elements consecutively, then uses a table of random numbers to draw the sample
    3. Using this technique eliminates the possibility of researcher bias and guarantees that differences in sample characteristics are attributable to chance
    4. Using this technique does not necessarily guarantee that the sample will be representative; however, the probability of choosing a nonrepresentative sample decreases as the sample size increases
    5. Researchers rarely use this technique because it is time-consuming and inefficient and because obtaining a complete listing of every element in a population may be impossible

C. Stratified random sampling
    1. *Stratified random sampling* involves the random selection of elements from two or more strata of the population to obtain a greater degree of representativeness
    2. When using this technique, the researcher must divide the population into homogeneous strata, then randomly select the sample following the same steps used in simple random sampling (see above)
    3. Using this technique guarantees the representation of different segments of the population and allows the researcher to oversample from a small stratum to adjust for its underrepresentation in the population
    4. Using stratified random sampling may be time-consuming, and the researcher may have difficulty establishing a stratified sampling frame that includes all the necessary elements

D. Cluster (multi-stage) sampling
    1. *Cluster sampling* involves the random sampling of elements from large groups (CLUSTERS) to successively smaller groups to narrow the sample to the smallest grouping possible

2. Typically, the researcher proceeds from the largest cluster (such as U.S. states) to progressively smaller clusters (such as counties, voting districts, and households) to arrive at the smallest element possible (such as male heads of households)

3. Cluster sampling is more economical and practical than simple or stratified random techniques, but it typically results in more sampling errors

E. Systematic sampling

1. *Systematic sampling* involves the random selection of subjects from the population based on a fixed SAMPLING INTERVAL (such as every 10th person in the sampling frame)

2. Most researchers prefer systematic sampling over simple random sampling because they can obtain the same results more efficiently and conveniently

3. Use of this technique may result in problems or questionable findings if the sampling frame is arranged so that a particular characteristic coincides with the sampling interval (for example, if every 10th person listed in the sampling frame is male)

III. Nonprobability (nonrandom) sampling

A. General information

1. Nonprobability sampling involves the selection of elements from a population using nonrandom procedures

2. Nonprobability sampling techniques are typically less rigorous and less representative than probability sampling techniques

3. Most research samples are based on nonprobability sampling because these techniques are feasible, practical, and relatively inexpensive

4. The major disadvantage to using nonprobability sampling is the researcher's limited ability to generalize from the findings

5. Nonprobability sampling can be further classified into four types: accidental (convenience), quota, purposive (judgmental), and network (snowball)

B. Accidental (convenience) sampling

1. *Accidental sampling* involves the nonrandom selection of subjects based on their availability or convenient accessibility

2. Although easy to obtain, they are considered the weakest type of samples

3. Use of this technique may result in questionable findings, because the most available subjects may not be typical of the population in terms of the variables of interest

4. With accidental sampling, the risk of researcher bias is great and external validity is compromised

C. Quota sampling
   1. *Quota sampling* involves the nonrandom selection of elements based on the identification of specific characteristics to increase the sample's representativeness
   2. Similar to stratified random sampling, quota sampling is based on the identification of certain strata within the population and the proportional representation of each of those strata in the sample
   3. Quota sampling helps to address the overrepresentation and underrepresentation of certain elements in the population
   4. This technique contains an unknown degree of bias that affects external validity

D. Purposive (judgmental) sampling
   1. *Purposive sampling* involves the nonrandom selection of elements based on the researcher's judgment and knowledge about the population
   2. Purposive sampling is useful when a group of subjects is needed to participate in a pretest of newly developed instruments or when a group of experts is desirable to validate research information
   3. With purposive sampling, the risk of conscious and unconscious bias is great and the researcher's ability to generalize from the findings is limited

E. Network (snowball) sampling
   1. Network sampling involves the nonrandom selection of elements based on social networks
   2. When the researcher has found one subject who meets the criteria, that person is asked to help recruit or locate other subjects
   3. This technique is used to obtain subjects difficult to locate, such as alcoholics, drug abusers, and criminals
   4. With network sampling, the risk of bias is great because the subjects know each other

Points to remember

A population is the entire group of elements that meets the eligibility criteria; a sample is the subset of elements from the population being studied.

Generally, the larger the sample, the more representative it will be of the population.

A power analysis is typically the most accurate way to determine sample size.

Simple random, stratified random, cluster, and systematic sampling are types of probability sampling techniques.

Accidental, quota, purposive, and network sampling are types of nonprobability sampling techniques.

Nonprobability sampling techniques typically are more feasible, practical, and economical than probability sampling techniques but result in less representative samples.

Glossary

The following terms are defined in Appendix A, page 111.

cluster	power analysis
element	random
heterogeneity	sampling interval
homogeneity	

Study questions

To evaluate your understanding of this chapter, answer the following questions in the space provided; then compare your responses with the correct answers in Appendix B, page 117.

1. What is a population? _____

   _____

   _____

2. What is the difference between probability and nonprobability sampling

   techniques? _____

   _____

3. What are four types of probability sampling? _____

   _____

   _____

4. What are four types of nonprobability sampling? _____

   _____

   _____

CHAPTER 9

Data Collection Methods and Measurement Techniques

Learning objectives

Check off the following items once you've mastered them:

☐ Define *data collection*.

☐ Identify the various methods used to collect data.

☐ Describe three types of instrument reliability (stability, internal consistency, and equivalence) and four types of instrument validity (content, concurrent, predictive, and construct).

☐ Define *measurement*.

☐ Differentiate among the four levels of measurement: nominal, ordinal, interval, and ratio.

☐ Compare and contrast the advantages and disadvantages of each data collection method.

☐ State the criteria for critiquing data collection methods and measurement techniques.

I. Introduction

A. *Data collection* is the process by which the researcher acquires subjects and collects the information needed to answer the research problem

B. Data collection allows the researcher to measure the variables in the study

C. Before collecting the data, the researcher must make a number of decisions
   1. Which data to collect
   2. How to collect the data
   3. Who will collect the data
   4. Where to collect the data
   5. When to collect the data

D. The researcher may use various data collection methods to gather information, such as questionnaires, interviews, scales, observation, physiological measures, projective techniques, or the Delphi technique

E. The researcher should base the selection of a data collection method on three concerns
   1. The identified hypothesis or research problem
   2. The research design
   3. The amount of information already known about the variables

F. The device used to collect the data is referred to as an *instrument* or a *tool*
   1. Instruments facilitate variable observation and measurement
   2. The researcher may rely on an existing instrument or may develop a new one to fit the study's needs
      a. Instrument development requires a high degree of research expertise, because the instrument must be reliable and valid
         (1) *Reliability* refers to the degree of consistency and accuracy with which an instrument measures a variable
         (2) *Validity* refers to the extent to which an instrument measures what it is designed to measure
         (3) An unreliable instrument cannot be valid, but a reliable instrument can be invalid
      b. An instrument is considered highly reliable if it demonstrates little variation with repeated measurements and has a high TRUE SCORE (little measurement error)
         (1) An instrument's reliability can be further defined according to its stability, internal consistency, and equivalence
            (a) *Stability* refers to the extent to which the same results are obtained with repeated use of an instrument
            (b) *Internal consistency* refers to the extent to which all parts of an instrument measure the same variable

       (c) *Equivalence* refers to the extent to which different
          observers or different forms of an instrument yield the
          same results
  (2) An instrument's validity can be further classified as content,
     concurrent, predictive, or construct
      (a) *Content validity* refers to the extent to which an
         instrument measures the variable's expected content; the
         researcher typically verifies content validity by conducting
         a literature review to determine which content should be
         covered and by asking experts to evaluate the instrument's
         representativeness of the content
      (b) *Concurrent validity* refers to the extent to which an
         instrument can accurately identify subjects who differ with
         respect to a given characteristic; the researcher typically
         validates concurrent validity by using the instrument in
         conjunction with a second instrument already known to
         be valid
      (c) *Predictive validity* refers to the extent to which an
         instrument can accurately forecast characteristics; the
         researcher typically validates predictive validity by using
         the instrument, then comparing the results with some
         future outcome
      (d) *Construct validity* refers to the extent to which an
         individual actually possesses the characteristic being
         measured by the instrument; the researcher typically
         validates construct validity by using the KNOWN-GROUPS
         TECHNIQUE

II. Measurement techniques

A. General information
  1. *Measurement* integral to quantitative research is the process by which
     the researcher assigns specific numbers to the collected data
  2. The researcher measures each variable of the collected data according
     to its magnitude or quantity
  3. Measurements are made based on two assumptions
    a. Everything exists in some amount, which can be measured
    b. Attributes of an object vary and the variability can be expressed as
      a number that indicates how much of the attribute is present
  4. The researcher may use one of four levels of measurement (nominal,
     ordinal, interval, or ratio) when collecting data
  5. The researcher should always aim for the highest level of measurement
     possible; generally, the higher the level, the more information is
     available for analysis
    a. Data measured at one level may be downgraded to a lower level,
      but never advanced to a higher level

       b. The level of measurement affects the types of statistical analyses that can be performed on the collected data

B. Nominal level

    1. With the *nominal level* (the lowest level), the researcher assigns numbers to categorize specific characteristics of a variable (for example, in relation to marital status, 0 might represent single and 1, married)

    2. The numbers do not have any quantitative meaning and cannot be manipulated mathematically

    3. The amount in each category can be counted and occurrence can be determined

    4. Examples of nominal-level variables are gender, marital status, health status, and nursing specialty

C. Ordinal level

    1. With the *ordinal level* (the second lowest level), the researcher assigns numbers to categories and sorts variables based on their relative rank

    2. The intervals between the categories are not considered equal

    3. The numbers have some quantitative meaning and can be manipulated mathematically but only to a limited degree

    4. Examples of ordinal-level variables are ranking of height (tallest to shortest) and pain intensity (mild, moderate, or severe)

D. Interval level

    1. With the *interval level* (the second highest level), the researcher assigns numbers to categories and ranks the variables according to equally spaced intervals

    2. Interval-level measures do not have an ABSOLUTE ZERO POINT

    3. The possibility of mathematical manipulations is greatly increased; addition and subtraction can be meaningfully calculated

    4. Examples of interval-level variables are Fahrenheit and centigrade temperatures and anxiety levels measured on a Likert scale

E. Ratio level

    1. With the *ratio level* (the highest level), the researcher not only assigns numbers to categories and ranks the variables according to equally spaced intervals as in interval-level measurement, but also designates an absolute, meaningful zero

    2. All mathematical manipulations, such as addition, subtraction, multiplication, and division, can be calculated

    3. Examples of ratio-level variables are height, weight, time, and length

F. Measurement error

    1. All measurements used in data collection are fallible; all results have some degree of error

    2. All measured results contain a true score and an error component

        a. The *true score* is the value that would be obtained if the measurement instrument were perfect

        b. The *error component* is the difference between the true score and the measured score

    3. Measurement error is the result of extraneous factors that distort the measured score

III. Questionnaires and interviews

A. General information
    1. Questionnaires and interviews are the most commonly used data collection methods in nursing research
    2. Questions may be either closed-ended or open-ended
        a. CLOSED-ENDED QUESTIONS allow the subjects to choose appropriate answers from a predetermined list of responses; such questions facilitate analysis and ensure comparability of responses; although they are easy to administer, they are difficult to construct
        b. OPEN-ENDED QUESTIONS allow the subjects to respond in their own words; although they typically provide detailed information, they are time-consuming and sometimes difficult to analyze

B. Types of questionnaires and interviews
    1. The questionnaire or interview schedule may be highly structured, totally unstructured, or semistructured
    2. A *highly structured* questionnaire or interview schedule contains only predetermined questions and response options; subjects are asked to respond to the same questions in the same order, using the same set of response options
    3. In a *totally unstructured* questionnaire or interview schedule, the researcher collects data with no preconceived plan of content or order of information to obtain; subjects are simply encouraged to relate their experiences
    4. *Semistructured* questionnaires and interview schedules contain some open-ended questions and some closed-ended questions, and a specific format for obtaining the information is followed

C. Advantages of questionnaires and interviews
    1. Questionnaires are relatively efficient data collection methods in terms of money, time, and ease of administration
    2. Questionnaires offer the possibility of subjects' anonymity
    3. Interviews are associated with a high response rate and can be used with most subjects
    4. Interviews allow the researcher to observe the subjects while they respond to questions, which may lead to more information

D. Disadvantages of questionnaires and interviews
    1. Questionnaires may have a low response rate because the subjects can disregard or ignore the questionnaire

2. Questionnaires require subjects' ability to read, write, and comprehend questions to avoid misinterpretation
3. Interviews require considerable time and money and cannot offer subjects anonymity
4. Interviews introduce the possibility of bias because of interviewer-subject interaction
5. The reliability and validity of questionnaires and interviews depend on subjects' honest responses

IV. Scales

A. General information
   1. A scale is a commonly used data collection method in which the researcher asks subjects to rank variables on a continuum; it allows the researcher to distinguish quantitatively among subjects who differ with respect to the variables of interest
   2. Researchers typically use scales to measure psychosocial variables, such as self-concept, personality traits, and attitudes

B. Types of scales
   1. *Rating scales* require subjects to rate or rank a phenomenon at some point along a continuum that has been assigned a numerical value (for example, subjects might be asked to rate an object on a scale of 1 to 10, with 10 being the highest score)
   2. *Likert scales,* the most commonly used scales in nursing research, are designed to elicit opinions or attitudes; subjects are asked to indicate how strongly they agree or disagree with a series of statements based on a 4- to 7-point scale
   3. The *semantic differential scale* is used to measure attitudes or beliefs
      a. It consists of two opposite adjectives (such as "important" and "unimportant," or "weak" and "strong"), with a 7-point scale between them
      b. Subjects are asked to indicate the one point on the scale that describes their view of a variable of interest
   4. *Guttman scales* consist of a group of four or five statements with which the subject is asked to agree or disagree; the statements relate to only one variable and are arranged in a hierarchy, so that the subject who agrees with the strongest statement of the group will probably agree with all of the other statements on the scale
   5. *The visual analog scale* uses a 100-mm-long line that lists variable extremes (such as "best" and "worst") at each end of the line
      a. Subjects are asked to trace through the line to indicate the intensity of the variable
      b. The researcher then uses a ruler to measure from the left end of the line to the subject's mark to obtain the measured value

C. Advantages of scales
 1. Scales are an efficient way to measure quantitatively the degree or magnitude of specific variables
 2. The researcher can use scales for group and individual comparisons
 3. Scales can be administered orally or in writing
 4. Scales can be rigorously evaluated

D. Disadvantages of scales
 1. Scales are susceptible to *social desirability response-set bias*, the tendency to give an answer that is consistent with current social views
 2. Scales are susceptible to *extreme response-set bias*, the tendency to express an attitude at the extreme (such as "strongly agree")
 3. Scales are susceptible to *acquiescence response-set bias*, the tendency to always agree with statements regardless of their content

V. Observation

A. General information
 1. Observation can be used in both quantitative and qualitative research designs but is most commonly used in qualitative studies
 2. Although observation tends to be more subjective than other data collection methods, it is sometimes the only means of collecting data
 3. The researcher uses several techniques when defining which observations to record, how they will be recorded, and the frequency with which they will be recorded, including category systems, checklists, rating scales, time sampling, and event sampling
  a. A *category system* is a list to which all observations can be assigned; the categories are carefully defined and should be mutually exclusive
  b. A *checklist*, which may be used in conjunction with a category system, involves placing a tally mark on the data collection form each time the behavior is observed
  c. *Rating scales* (see above) can be used with a checklist to indicate the magnitude or intensity of the observed behavior
  d. *Time sampling* involves the selection of periods during which the observation will occur (such as every 2 minutes for 15 seconds)
  e. *Event sampling* involves the selection of specific events to observe (such as shift changes or medication administration)

B. Types of observation
 1. *Unstructured* or PARTICIPANT OBSERVATION, used in qualitative research (particularly ethnography), involves the researcher in the study to gain information that might otherwise be missed; typically, the researcher compiles voluminous narrative data, using logs and field notes

2. *Structured* observation involves precise record-keeping methods (such as category systems, checklists, and rating scales) to record observations accurately; the researcher typically has some prior knowledge about the behavior or event of interest

C. Advantages of observation
1. Observation can be used effectively in many types of research studies
2. Observation allows the researcher to see behaviors and events firsthand and to take detailed notes
3. Unstructured observation is inherently flexible and allows the researcher to reconceptualize the problem after becoming more familiar with the circumstances

D. Disadvantages of observation
1. Subjects who are aware of being observed may behave atypically, which may threaten the study's validity
2. The use of subjects who are unaware of being observed may be unethical
3. The data are subject to observer distortion and bias

VI. Physiological measures

A. General information
1. Physiological measures, the collection of information on physical variables, has become increasingly popular because of recent interest in clinical research
2. Physiological measures have been used to study body processes, ways in which nursing actions affect outcomes, effectiveness of nursing interventions, and ways to improve the measuring and recording of physiological information
3. Many physiological measures require specific instrumentation

B. Types of physiological measures
1. *Direct* methods use straightforward techniques to measure the variable, such as using a thermometer to measure temperature
2. *Indirect* methods use indirect techniques that are conceptually linked to the framework to measure the variable, such as using heart rate and blood pressure to measure anxiety

C. Advantages of physiological measures
1. Physiological measures are objective and tend to be precise and accurate
2. Subjects are less likely to distort measurements deliberately
3. Because the instruments are designed to measure physiological data, validity is assumed
4. Most of the necessary equipment for collecting data is available in hospitals

CHECKLIST: DATA COLLECTION METHODS AND MEASUREMENT TECHNIQUES

Use the following questions to critique the data collection method used in a study.

	Yes	No
General questions		
• Is the data collection method clearly described?	☐	☐
• Is the appropriate method used for the research design and the population?	☐	☐
• Is the same data collection method used for all subjects?	☐	☐
• Does the researcher discuss the reliability and validity of the method used?	☐	☐
Questionnaires and interviews		
• Is the degree of structure consistent with the research question?	☐	☐
• Did the researcher use the appropriate method (questionnaire vs. interview) for the research design?	☐	☐
• Is the questionnaire or interview schedule sufficiently described to determine whether it covers the variable of interest?	☐	☐
• Did sufficient numbers of subjects respond?	☐	☐
• If an interview was used, were the interviewers trained?	☐	☐
Scales		
• Does the scale adequately cover the variables?	☐	☐
• Did the researcher use the most appropriate scale for collecting the data?	☐	☐
• If the researcher used a new scale, was it adequately pretested and refined?	☐	☐
• Does the researcher address the possibility of response-set biases?	☐	☐
Observation		
• Is the degree of structure imposed by the researcher consistent with the research question?	☐	☐
• Were the observers required to make any judgments about what they observed?	☐	☐
• Was an appropriate category system, checklist, or rating scale used?	☐	☐
• Did the observer's presence affect the subjects' behavior?	☐	☐
• If time sampling or event sampling was used, did the sampling plan yield relevant behaviors?	☐	☐

(continued)

CHECKLIST: DATA COLLLECTION METHODS AND MEASUREMENT TECHNIQUES
(continued)

Physiological measures	Yes	No
• Was the proper instrument used to obtain the measurements?	☐	☐
• If an invasive procedure was used, could a noninvasive procedure have yielded similar information?	☐	☐
• Did the instrument appear to have any effect on the variable being measured?	☐	☐
• Was the instrument reliable and valid for the variable of interest?	☐	☐
Delphi technique		
• Were the panel members experts on the variable of interest?	☐	☐
• Did the study suffer from severe attrition of panel members?	☐	☐
• Were enough rounds of questionnaires, analysis, and feedback completed?	☐	☐
• Was a consensus reached?	☐	☐

D. Disadvantages of physiological data measures
1. The instrument itself may affect the variable being measured
2. Electrical interferences in the instrument may create measurement distortions
3. The researcher must be especially careful to prevent injury to subjects whenever high levels of energy are required to take measurements
4. The researcher may need specialized knowledge and preparation to use the equipment
5. Instrument calibration is necessary to ensure accuracy

VII. Delphi technique

A. General information
1. The Delphi technique collects opinions from various experts on a variable of interest without the need for a joint panel discussion
2. The researcher identifies and selects a panel of experts
   a. They are asked to complete a questionnaire on the variable
   b. After analyzing the data, the researcher returns the results to the experts along with a second questionnaire that, when completed, is to be returned to the researcher for analysis
   c. The experts are allowed to reformulate opinions based on the feedback received after each questionnaire

      d. The questionnaire-analysis cycle may be continued three to five times or until a consensus is reached; extending the cycle beyond five times increases the risk of subject attrition from the experts' growing disinterest in the study

B. Advantages of the Delphi technique
    1. The Delphi technique is an effective and efficient means of obtaining the opinions of a large group of experts
    2. Any one persuasive expert cannot unduly influence the group's opinions
    3. Anonymity may encourage honest opinions

C. Disadvantages of the Delphi technique
    1. The Delphi technique is expensive and time-consuming because of repeated collection and analysis
    2. Because panel members may become uncooperative if the study does not progress swiftly, an adequate sample may be difficult to maintain (see *Checklist: Data Collection Methods and Measurement Techniques,* pages 86 and 87)

Points to remember

Data collection and measurement can provide the researcher with the information needed to answer the research problem.

The four levels of measurement are nominal, ordinal, interval, and ratio.

The researcher should never design a study to fit an instrument, select an instrument that has little relationship to the theoretical framework, or use an instrument without first examining its reliability and validity.

The types of reliability associated with instrument measurement are stability, internal consistency, and equivalence.

The types of validity involved in instrument measurement are content, concurrent, predictive, and construct.

Questionnaires and interviews are the most commonly used data collection methods in nursing research.

Observation, which is most frequently used in qualitative studies, tends to be more subjective than other data collection methods.

Physiological measures usually require instrumentation and tend to be more objective than other data collection methods.

Glossary

The following terms are defined in Appendix A, page 111.

absolute zero point	open-ended question
closed-ended question	participant observation
known-groups technique	true score

Study questions

To evaluate your understanding of this chapter, answer the following questions in the space provided; then compare your responses with the correct answers in Appendix B, page 117.

1. What are three types of reliability? _____

   _____

   _____

2. What are four types of validity? _____

   _____

   _____

3. What are the four levels of measurement, from lowest to highest? _____

   _____

   _____

4. What are the most commonly used data collection methods? _____

   _____

   _____

5. What is the main disadvantage of questionnaires? _____

   _____

6. What is the main advantage of a scale? _____

   _____

   _____

7. What is the main advantage of physiological data collection measures?

   _____

   _____

CHAPTER 10

Data Analysis

Learning objectives

Check off the following items once you've mastered them:

☐ State the purpose of data analysis.

☐ Identify the ways in which computers are used in quantitative data analysis.

☐ Describe four categories of descriptive statistics: frequency distribution, measures of central tendency, measures of variability, and bivariate.

☐ List 14 frequently used inferential statistical tests: *t*-test, analysis of variance, chi-square analysis, Mann-Whitney *U*, Kruskal-Wallis, Wilcoxon signed-rank, correlation coefficient, simple linear regression, multiple regression, canonical correlation, analysis of covariance, multivariate analysis of variance, discriminant analysis, and path analysis.

☐ Explain the constant comparative method, content analysis, analytical induction, and hermeneutical analysis.

☐ State the criteria for critiquing quantitative and qualitative data analysis.

I. Introduction

A. Data analysis involves various techniques to summarize and examine the collected information to help determine trends and relationships among the variables

B. Its primary purpose is to impose order on voluminous data so that conclusions can be made and communicated

C. The research design dictates which techniques should be used to analyze the data
   1. Quantitative research designs use numbers and statistical techniques
   2. Qualitative research designs use words and logic

II. Quantitative data analysis

A. General information
   1. Quantitative data analysis involves the use of statistical computations to summarize the collected data, compare and contrast the data, test theoretical relationships, generalize about the population based on sample findings, and evaluate cause-and-effect relationships
   2. Most researchers rely on computers to help with computations
   3. Computers also help the researcher to detect data coding and entry errors, edit and sort the data, merge data from two or more sources into one data file, store the data for retrieval, and display the data in table or graph form
   4. Statistical packages available for computer quantitative data analysis include Statistical Packages for the Social Sciences, Statistical Analysis System, and Biomedical Data Programs
   5. The researcher performs statistical computations for each hypothesis or research question; the statistics used may be descriptive or inferential
      a. Descriptive statistics summarize the data and describe sample characteristics
      b. Inferential statistics enable the researcher to generalize about the population based on data obtained from the sample

B. Descriptive statistics
   1. *Descriptive* (or *summary*) *statistics* are numerical values obtained from a sample that provide some meaning or insight into the characteristics
   2. All quantitative data analyses begin with descriptive statistics
      a. The extent to which the researcher relies on descriptive statistics depends on the type of research design
      b. For example, in exploratory or descriptive research designs, descriptive statistics are typically the only statistics used for data analysis; in other research designs, descriptive statistics are typically used to summarize the sample characteristics

3. Descriptive statistics can be classified into four categories: frequency distributions, measures of central tendency, measures of variability, and bivariate descriptive statistics

   a. *Frequency distribution* is the arrangement of all numerical values assigned to variables, from the lowest to the highest, along with a listing of the number of times each value was obtained; this arrangement is a useful way of organizing and summarizing data and can be used for analysis

     (1) Frequency distributions can be ungrouped (each value is listed separately) or grouped (values are organized according to ranges or intervals)

     (2) Frequency distributions may be displayed in table or graph form (see *Frequency Distributions: Tables and Graphs*, page 94)

     (3) When represented in graph form, frequency distributions are typically described in terms of their curved shape

       (a) They may be symmetrical (consisting of identical halves) or asymmetrical (containing off-center peaks and unequal sides or tails; asymmetrical curves, also known as skewed curves, can be positively or negatively skewed, depending on the direction in which the tail is pointing)

       (b) They may be unimodal (containing only one peak) or multimodal (containing two or more peaks)

       (c) A normal distribution curve (depicted by a bell-shaped curve that is symmetrical, unimodal, and not too peaked) represents the normal variations of a variable within a given population (50% of the values lie on the right half of the curve and 50% lie on the left half)

   b. *Measures of central tendency* are statistics that summarize the data into one representative value; they include the mode, the median, and the mean

     (1) The *mode* is the score or category that has the highest frequency or that occurs most often on a frequency distribution; it is typically used with nominal-level measures

     (2) The *median* is the number that lies midpoint in a distribution and divides the scores in half; because of its insensitivity to extreme values, the median is commonly the preferred measure of central tendency when the distribution is skewed

     (3) The *mean* is the arithmetic average of a distribution that can be used with only interval or ratio data; the mean, which is commonly symbolized as $\overline{X}$ or M, is the most commonly used measure of central tendency and the least likely to fluctuate widely from one sample to another sample drawn from the same population

FREQUENCY DISTRIBUTIONS: TABLES AND GRAPHS

A frequency distribution—a systematic arrangement of numerical values, from the lowest to the highest, coupled with a tally of the number of times each value was obtained—may be illustrated in the form of a table or graph. Below are examples of various frequency distributions representing the raw test scores of a group of 50 students whose scores ranged from 20 to 30.

FREQUENCY TABLE

Raw scores	Tallies	Frequency	Percentage (%)
20	I I I I	4	8.0
21	I I I	3	6.0
22	I I I I	4	8.0
23	I I I I I	5	10.0
24	I I I I I I I I I	9	18.0
25	I I I I I I I	7	14.0
26	I I I I I I	6	12.0
27	I I I I	4	8.0
28	I I I	3	6.0
29	I I I	3	6.0
30	I I	2	4.0

HISTOGRAM

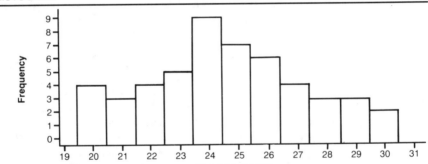

FREQUENCY POLYGON

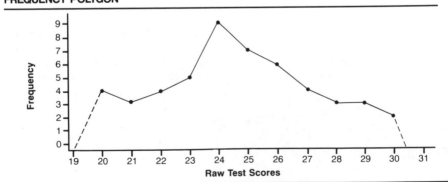

c. *Measures of variability* are statistics that concern the degree to which the scores in a distribution are different from or similar to each other; the two most commonly used are the range and the standard deviation
  (1) The *range* is the distance between the highest score and the lowest score in a distribution
  (2) The *standard deviation* is the most commonly used measure of variability; it indicates the average to which scores deviate from the mean; the standard deviation, commonly symbolized as *SD*, is an indication of the degree of error involved when the mean is used to describe a distribution
  (3) A normal distribution contains approximately three standard deviations above and below the mean; about 68% of all scores fall within one standard deviation of the mean, about 95% fall within two standard deviations of the mean, and about 99% fall within three standard deviations of the mean
d. *Bivariate (two-variable) descriptive statistics* are those derived from the simultaneous analysis of two variables to examine the relationships between the variables; the two most commonly used in quantitative analysis are contingency tables and correlation
  (1) A *contingency table* allows the visual comparison of two or more categories of nominal- or ordinal-level data; typically, the data are in the form of numbers or percentages that appear within individual table cells
  (2) *Correlation* involves the use of a correlation coefficient (ranging from $+1.00$ to -1.00) to describe the relationship between two variables
    (a) A correlation coefficient of 0 indicates that no relationship exists between the two variables
    (b) A correlation coefficient between 0 and $+1.00$ indicates a positive relationship (as one variable increases, the other variable also increases)
    (c) A correlation coefficient between 0 and -1.00 indicates a negative or inverse relationship (as one variable increases, the other variable decreases)
    (d) The higher the absolute value of the coefficient, the stronger the relationship (for example, -0.75 indicates a stronger relationship than $+0.25$)
    (e) The *product moment correlation coefficient,* known as the PEARSON *r,* is the most commonly used correlation procedure involving interval- or ratio-level data
C. Inferential statistics
  1. *Inferential statistics* are numerical values used to draw conclusions about a population based on the characteristics of a population sample
  2. Inferential statistics are based on the laws of probability

---

CHECKLIST: QUANTITATIVE DATA ANALYSIS

Use the following questions to critique the quantitative data analysis used in a study.

	Yes	No
• Does the research question or hypothesis lend itself to quantitative analysis?	☐	☐
• Was the level of measurement appropriate for the data collection tool?	☐	☐
• Were the statistical tests appropriate for the level of measurement?	☐	☐
• Have all frequencies, measures of central tendency, and measures of variability been reported?	☐	☐
• Was a statistical test performed for each research question or hypothesis?	☐	☐
• Did the researcher select an appropriate level of significance?	☐	☐
• If a parametric test was used, were the data measured on an interval or a ratio level? Were the variables normally distributed throughout the population?	☐	☐
• If a nonparametric test was used, could the researcher have used a more powerful parametric test?	☐	☐
• Did the researcher present a sufficient amount of information about the analyzed data and results to support the hypothesis or research question?	☐	☐
• Did the researcher use frequency distribution tables or graphs to summarize large amounts of data? Are they clearly labeled and consistent with the text?	☐	☐

---

3. The underlying assumption is that only chance is responsible for variation among samples of the same population

4. Inferential statistics provide objective criteria for deciding whether a hypothesis should be accepted as true or rejected as false and for deciding which outcomes probably resulted from chance

5. An important factor in determining the degree to which chance affects the findings is the level of significance the researcher assigns to the findings

   a. The *level of significance* is a numerical value selected by the researcher before data collection to indicate the probability of erroneous findings being accepted as true; this value typically is represented as 0.01 or 0.05

    b. A 0.05 level of significance indicates that of 100 samples, the researcher would expect 5 samples to yield erroneous findings and 95 samples to yield accurate findings; a 0.01 level of significance indicates that of 100 samples, the researcher would expect 1 sample to yield erroneous findings and 99 samples to yield accurate findings

6. Inferential statistical tests can be classified according to two types: parametric and nonparametric; parametric tests are more powerful and flexible than nonparametric tests and are preferred by most researchers

    a. *Parametric* tests focus on population parameters, require measurements on an interval or ratio level, and assume that the variables are normally distributed in the population

    b. *Nonparametric* tests are not based on population parameters, use nominal- or ordinal-level data, and assume nothing about the distribution of the variables in the population

7. The most commonly used inferential statistical tests include the *t*-test, analysis of variance, chi-square analysis, Mann-Whitney *U*, Kruskal-Wallis, Wilcoxon signed-rank, correlation coefficient, simple linear regression, multiple regression, canonical correlation, analysis of covariance, multivariate analysis of variance, discriminant analysis, and path analysis (see *Checklist: Quantitative Data Analysis*)

III. Qualitative data analysis

A. General information

1. Qualitative data analysis relies on intuition and analytical reasoning to guide the organization, reduction, and clustering of data

2. The researcher typically uses three strategies to analyze the data

    a. *Reduction* is the minute examination of voluminous narrative data that allows the researcher to deduce inherent meanings

    b. *Data display* is the organization of data using tables, graphs, and matrices

    c. *Conclusion drawing and verification* is the process whereby the researcher attaches meaning to the findings

3. Many researchers use computers to help with data analysis

4. Computer programs available for analysis of qualitative data include Ethnograph, Superfile, TEXTAN, Framework, and Quad

5. Qualitative data analysis is particularly challenging for three reasons

    a. The researcher has no systematic rules to guide the analysis and interpretation of data

    b. The researcher must devote much time and work to reading, organizing, and analyzing the data

    c. The findings cannot be briefly summarized (in fact, many analyses are published as books rather than as research articles)

6. The researcher must develop an effective record-keeping and data retrieval system, either manually or on computer, in which all data are labeled, indexed, sorted, and filed
7. The researcher may use one of four methods to conduct qualitative data analysis: the constant comparative method, content analysis, analytical induction, or hermeneutical analysis

B. Constant comparative method
   1. The *constant comparative method* is a means of analyzing data collected through grounded theory, in which the researcher collects and analyzes data simultaneously without the use of a pre-existing theory as an organizing framework
   2. In this type of analysis, which typically requires considerable time and the ability to think conceptually, the researcher attempts to discover patterns or social behaviors to form the basis of a relevant and useful theory that has the potential for generalizability
   3. To conduct a constant comparative analysis, the researcher first formulates a research question, then uses theoretical sampling to obtain data from various subjects and situations
   4. After obtaining the data, the researcher takes the following steps
      a. Establishes categories or codes based on the similarity or dissimilarity of the content
      b. Compares each incident with the category to determine if each incident fits
      c. Examines categories for uniformities and differences
      d. Reviews the literature to discover how the current research fits with existing research
      e. Discovers the overriding conceptual scheme that accounts for most of the relationships or patterns observed
      f. Sorts the data into a coherent whole that integrates all of the main ideas into a scheme
      g. Writes a report

C. Content analysis
   1. *Content analysis* involves the systematic and objective quantification of data to analyze the content of individual words, phrases, sentences, or themes
   2. Used with either oral or written data, content analysis is especially useful in historical research because of the efficient manner in which materials are used
   3. The researcher strives to maintain objectivity by having two people analyze the same data
   4. To conduct a content analysis, the researcher takes the following steps
      a. Identifies and selects the variables or concepts to be recorded and the unit of analysis (the word, phrase, sentence, or theme) to be used

---

CHECKLIST: QUALITATIVE DATA ANALYSIS

Use the following questions to critique the qualitative data analysis used in a study.

	Yes	No
• Was qualitative analysis appropriate for the research question and design?	☐	☐
• If any of the qualitative data were converted to quantitative data, was the level of quantification appropriate?	☐	☐
• Were the sources of data (such as observations or interviews) sufficient to yield a broad range of material for analysis?	☐	☐
• Did the researcher provide excerpts from the narrative material to demonstrate and substantiate the themes identified in the data?	☐	☐
• Did the researcher search for negative cases?	☐	☐
• Is the researcher's attempt to be objective evident?	☐	☐

---

   b. Formulates a coding and category system for classifying the units
      of analysis
   c. Develops definitions and illustrations to guide the coding of data
      into categories
   d. Analyzes the data by counting the coded information
   e. Draws conclusions
   f. Issues a report of the findings

D. Analytical induction
   1. *Analytical induction* involves searching for concepts and propositions
      in data that are applicable to all cases of the topic of interest or
      question being studied
   2. The researcher must carefully consider all aspects of the data, analyze
      each case separately, and compare each case to the others
   3. To conduct analytical induction, the researcher takes the following
      steps
      a. Defines the phenomenon to be analyzed
      b. Reviews the data
      c. Formulates a hypothetical explanation of the phenomenon
      d. Examines each case to see if the hypothesis applies
      e. Searches for negative cases (situations for which the hypothesis
         does not apply)
      f. Reformulates the hypothesis, as necessary
      g. Continues examining cases and reformulating the hypothesis until
         a universal pattern of relationships is identified and supported by
         the data

E. Hermeneutical analysis

1. *Hermeneutical analysis,* sometimes called phenomenological-interpretive analysis, is a holistic approach to analysis that involves the examination and interpretation of field notes or interviews to understand the meanings and practices of people functioning as whole beings in specific situations

2. Hermeneutical analysis is based on three assumptions
   a. Language is used by individuals to communicate their ideas about reality
   b. The researcher's task is to uncover and understand the meanings embedded in communication
   c. The researcher must study normal activities of daily life

3. The researcher typically analyzes the data to identify which aspects of specific behaviors or situations are important to the subject and the specific meanings the subject attaches to them

4. The researcher may use one of three approaches to conducting hermeneutical analysis
   a. *Thematic analysis* involves reading each interview to identify common themes
   b. *Analysis of exemplars* involves examining events taken from interviews to generate descriptions of situations and behaviors
   c. *Identification of a* PARADIGM CASE involves examining all cases to find similarities between the paradigm and the other cases (see *Checklist: Qualitative Data Analysis,* page 99)

Points to remember

The purpose of data analysis is to impose order on a large amount of information so that conclusions can be made and communicated.

Computers can be widely used in data analysis and have almost eliminated the need for manual statistical computations.

Descriptive statistics include frequency distributions, measures of central tendency, measures of variability, and bivariate statistics.

Commonly used inferential statistical tests include the t-test, analysis of variance, chi-square, Mann-Whitney U, Kruskal-Wallis, Wilcoxon signed-rank, correlation coefficient, simple linear regression, multiple regression, canonical correlation, analysis of covariance, multivariate analysis of variance, discriminant analysis, and path analysis.

Qualitative data may be analyzed using the constant comparative method, content analysis, analytical induction, or hermeneutical analysis.

Glossary

The following terms are defined in Appendix A, page 111.

paradigm case

Pearson r

Study questions

To evaluate your understanding of this chapter, answer the following questions in the space provided; then compare your responses with the correct answers in Appendix B, pages 117 and 118.

1. What is the purpose of data analysis? _____

_____

_____

2. Which type of data analysis uses numbers and statistical computations?

_____

_____

3. Which type of data analysis uses words and analytical reasoning? _____

_____

_____

4. What are the four categories of descriptive statistics? _____

_____

_____

5. What methods might be used to analyze qualitative data? _____

_____

_____

CHAPTER 11

Interpretation, Communication, and Use of Research Findings

Learning objectives

Check off the following items once you've mastered them:

☐ Differentiate between statistical and clinical significance.

☐ Compare and contrast narrative and pictorial presentations of findings.

☐ Describe the relationship between findings and implications for nursing.

☐ Discuss oral, poster, and written formats used to communicate research findings.

☐ Identify barriers to using research.

☐ Discuss strategies for increasing the use of research.

☐ State the criteria for critiquing the research report.

I. Introduction

A. The INTERPRETATION and communication of findings are the final steps in the research process

B. The researcher relies on creativity, logical reasoning, intelligence, and communication skills to arrive at conclusions and issue a report of the findings

C. The report may be presented orally at a conference or in writing as a research article

II. Interpreting research findings

A. General information
   1. Interpretation is the process by which the researcher examines, organizes, and attaches significance to the results obtained from the data analysis
   2. The researcher typically relies on introspection, logic, and intuition
   3. The researcher should base the interpretation of findings on the problem statement, conceptual or theoretical framework, hypotheses or research questions, literature review, population studied, and limitations of the research design

B. Significance of the findings
   1. The researcher's interpretation of the data after analysis should yield one of three possible results: statistically significant findings that match the hypothesized findings, significant findings that contradict the hypothesized findings, or nonsignificant findings
      a. Statistically significant findings that match the hypothesized findings are typically the easiest to interpret because the researcher will have already examined the variables and predicted the results
      b. Significant findings that contradict the hypothesized findings may result from the researcher's faulty logic or from flaws within the theory itself
      c. Nonsignificant findings may result from inappropriate methodology, a biased or small sample, threats to internal validity, unreliable or invalid instruments, weak statistical measures, faulty analysis, or theoretical weaknesses
   2. The researcher must be especially careful to distinguish STATISTICAL SIGNIFICANCE from CLINICAL SIGNIFICANCE
      a. *Statistical significance* means that the null hypothesis has been rejected and any differences between groups are probably not the result of chance; statistical significance depends on sample size: the larger the sample, the greater the possibility of statistical significance
      b. *Clinical significance* means that the findings may be useful in a clinical setting

C. Presentation of the findings
    1. Findings usually are presented narratively and pictorially
        a. A narrative presentation, which typically constitutes the text portion of a written report, should include specific information on the statistical test used, the results, and the probability value
        b. A pictorial presentation typically includes illustrated graphs, HISTOGRAMS, pie charts, and FREQUENCY POLYGONS and tables
    2. Tables used to summarize findings should be clearly labeled with titles that accurately identify the variables being presented; numbers should be consistently rounded to the same number of decimal places, with all decimal points aligned
    3. When coordinating the narrative and illustrated portions of a report, the researcher should ensure that nothing in the text repeats what is in the illustrated portions and, conversely, that nothing in the illustrated portions repeats what is in the text

D. Forming conclusions
    1. The researcher deduces conclusions from the current study findings coupled with information learned in previous research studies
    2. When forming conclusions, the researcher must remember that research never proves anything — it merely lends support to a position
    3. The researcher must always guard against allowing subjective judgments and biases to creep into conclusions
    4. The researcher should also avoid extending conclusions beyond the available data

E. Nursing implications
    1. When formulating conclusions, the researcher must provide practical suggestions for implementing the findings in nursing
    2. The researcher must consider which areas of nursing may be affected by the study findings and include at least one nursing implication for each conclusion drawn
    3. Such implications typically focus on changes that should or should not be made in nursing practice, education, and research

III. Communicating research findings

A. General information
    1. The researcher must communicate findings to practitioners and researchers so that the study has an impact on nursing practice
    2. To communicate the findings, the researcher must develop a RESEARCH REPORT that clearly and concisely describes the research problem, methodology, findings, and interpretation of the findings
    3. The report may be written or presented orally or pictorially in poster form; usually, an oral report presented at a conference is the quickest means of communicating the findings (see *Checklist: Research Report*, page 106)

CHECKLIST: RESEARCH REPORT

Use the following questions as a guide to critiquing the research report of a study.

	Yes	No
• Considering the constraints on time and space, does the report include sufficient detail to permit a thorough critique of the study?	☐	☐
• Does the report include information on the research problem, framework, methodology, findings, and interpretation of the findings?	☐	☐
• Are tables and figures used to present the findings clearly titled and do they supplement the text?	☐	☐
• Is the report clear and concise?	☐	☐
• Is the report well organized and logically presented?	☐	☐
• Are implications for nursing practice, education, or research included in the conclusions?	☐	☐
• Does the researcher generalize about the results within the study's scope?	☐	☐

B. Oral reports
   1. Presenting an oral report at a conference enables the researcher to disseminate the information quickly and to interact directly with the conference participants; however, because the number of conference attendees is typically limited, the researcher's ability to share the findings with a wide audience is limited
   2. Most oral presentations are limited to approximately 20 minutes; therefore, the researcher typically needs to give a condensed report of the findings and eliminate many of the study's details
   3. The researcher may rely on slides or transparencies to enhance the presentation and use an informal, lively tone when speaking

C. Poster presentations
   1. Poster presentations have become an increasingly popular way to communicate findings
   2. The researcher should remain with the poster to talk with the viewers and answer questions
   3. The poster's appearance plays an important role in communicating the findings; it should incorporate color, diagrams, and graphs and should neatly and clearly present the content of the study in large, easy-to-read type

D. Written reports
   1. The researcher may choose to communicate the research findings through a written report

2. Submitting a report for publication in a journal enables the researcher to communicate more detailed information about the study to a wider audience; however, depending on when and if the manuscript is accepted for publication, months or years may elapse before the report is finally published and read
3. When writing a report, the researcher must keep in mind the intended audience and use of the report
   a. For example, a report intended for publication in a nursing journal should contain appropriate language and should be concisely written to the desired article length
   b. As another example, a report intended for submission as a thesis or dissertation should demonstrate an in-depth understanding of the subject and the research process
4. A well-written report, which typically traces the study from beginning to end, has several parts
   a. An introductory discussion of the research problem and rationale for conducting the study
   b. A review of the literature used to develop the study and the framework that guided the study
   c. A detailed explanation of the methodology used to conduct the study, including information on the specific research design, sampling technique, and data collection method
   d. A presentation of the results, including the data analysis used and the researcher's interpretation of the findings
   e. The researcher's conclusions about the research findings and their implications for nursing

IV. Using research findings

A. General information
   1. The ultimate value of nursing research is the extent to which it is used in practice
   2. The purpose of research use is to get the solutions identified through research used for the good of society

B. Barriers to research use
   1. The majority of practicing nurses have not received instruction in research and lack the skills to evaluate and critique research reports
   2. Several years may pass between the time a researcher designs a study and practicing nurses learn about the results
   3. Research reports may be seen as difficult to read and understand
   4. Individuals and organizations are usually reluctant to change
   5. Practicing nurses have not been rewarded for implementing research findings
   6. Resources may not be available for conducting research or implementing findings
   7. Researchers and practitioners fail to communicate and collaborate

C. Research use efforts
1. The Western Interstate Commission for Higher Education regional nursing research development project, initiated in the mid-1970s, was the first major effort focusing on nursing research use; nurses were given the opportunity to evaluate research aimed at solving practice problems
2. The Conduct and Utilization of Research in Nursing project, conducted from 1975 to 1980, sought to increase use of research findings by disseminating quality findings and facilitating their implementation
3. The Nursing Child Assessment Satellite Training project, begun in 1976, was educational and aimed at the practicing nurse; it supported the use of satellite communication for research dissemination
4. The Agency for Health Care Policy and Research of the U.S. Department of Health and Human Services' Public Health Service, in the early 1990s, developed clinical practice guidelines based on research

D. Strategies for increasing research use
1. Researchers should take the responsibility to conduct quality research in which the findings include clear implications for practice and are communicated clearly at every opportunity; researchers should also replicate studies and collaborate with practitioners
2. Educators should integrate research findings throughout the curriculum, stimulate intellectual curiosity and inquiry, and be actively involved in research activities
3. Administrators should offer emotional and financial support for efforts to use research and should reward its use
4. Practicing nurses should critically read research literature, attend professional meetings, collaborate with nursing researchers, and participate in research use projects

Points to remember

Interpretation of research findings requires the use of introspection, logical reasoning, and intuition.

Statistically significant findings suggest that differences between groups probably did not result from chance.

Clinically significant findings are useful in the practice setting.

All conclusions drawn from the findings should address the implications for nursing in relation to practice, education, and research.

Findings must be communicated to and implemented by practitioners for research to have an effect on nursing practice.

Research findings are typically communicated through a research report that may be written or presented orally or in poster form.

Narrative presentations are typically supplemented by illustrated tables and graphs.

Presenting a research report at a conference disseminates the findings rapidly; publishing a written report reaches a wider audience.

The ultimate value of research is the extent to which it is used in practice.

Glossary

The following terms are defined in Appendix A, page 111.

clinical significance   interpretation

frequency polygon   research report

histogram   statistical significance

Study questions

To evaluate your understanding of this chapter, answer the following questions in the space provided; then compare your responses with the correct answers in Appendix B, page 118.

1. What skills does the researcher use to interpret the findings? _____

   _____

   _____

2. What is the difference between statistical significance and clinical significance? _____

   _____

3. Why are nursing implications important? _____

   _____

   _____

4. What are three ways in which research findings might be communicated?

   _____

   _____

5. How might the practicing nurse increase research use? _____

   _____

   _____

Appendices

A: Glossary

Absolute zero point — point in measurement indicating a total absence of the item or attribute being measured; in interval level measurement, the zero point is arbitrary, not absolute

Abstract — brief summary of a research study

Clinical significance — usefulness of a study's findings in a clinical setting

Closed-ended question — one that limits the respondent to a fixed number of answer choices

Cluster — large grouping of elements within a population

Concept — term to which a label or meaning is attached

Conceptual framework — abstract organization of concepts that provides direction for a research study

Confidentiality — protection of personal information gathered against unnecessary divulgence

Database — large collection of information in a computer that can be rapidly retrieved and rearranged; listings may be updated regularly

Deductive reasoning — process by which specifics are inferred from general principles; relies on the accuracy of the general principles to arrive at valid conclusions

Descriptive research — study in which the researcher accurately portrays the characteristics of a particular individual, situation, or group to outline existence, determine the frequency with which something occurs, or classify information

Dissertation — original research study written by a candidate for a doctoral degree

Effect size — statistical expression describing the magnitude of a relationship between two variables

Element — basic unit that makes up the sample and the population about which information is collected

Empirical evidence — data based on objective observation or experience

Empirical testing — objective analysis, typically using statistical techniques, of evidence gained objectively through the senses

Exploratory research — preliminary study conducted to gain insight, discover ideas, or increase knowledge in a particular area

Frequency polygon — graphic representation of a frequency distribution that uses dots connected by straight lines to depict the frequency (number) of data identified on a horizontal axis

Hawthorne effect — effect on the dependent variable caused by the subjects' knowledge that they are participating in a research study

Heterogeneity — extent to which subjects in a sample are dissimilar in some specific way

Histogram — graphic representation of a frequency distribution that uses vertical bars to depict the frequency of data identified on a horizontal axis

Holism — philosophical view that an individual is more than the sum of his or her parts and must be studied as a whole

Homogeneity — extent to which subjects in a sample are similar in some specific way

Hypothesis — statement of a predicted relationship between the concepts examined in a study

Inductive reasoning — process by which general principles are inferred from specific observations; relies on the representativeness of the specific observations to arrive at valid conclusions

Informed consent — voluntary participation of subjects in a research study based on full understanding of the study before it begins

Institutional review board — committee established by an organization to evaluate all research conducted in that facility

Interpretation — process by which the results obtained from a data analysis are examined, organized, and assigned some significance

Known-groups technique—approach used to determine the construct validity of an instrument in which the researcher uses the instrument on two groups of subjects who are expected to differ with regard to a variable of interest (such as a group of depressed subjects and a group of nondepressed subjects) and then measures the differences to test the instrument's validity

Literature review—critical summary of research findings and theoretical information on a topic

Model—symbolic representation of a conceptual or theoretical framework that uses boxes, arrows, letters, numbers, or other symbols to convey meaning

Open-ended question—one that allows the respondent to answer in a narrative form, using his or her own words

Operational definition—actions or operations that the researcher must perform to measure a variable

Paradigm case—example that contains all of the critical elements demonstrating the situation being studied

Participant observation—unstructured method of collecting data about a group in which the researcher acts as a group member as well as an observer

Pearson *r*—mathematical computation used to compare the extent of a relationship between two variables

Pilot study—small-scale version of a proposed research study performed to refine methodology

Population—entire group of people or objects that a study covers

Power analysis—statistical procedure used to determine sample size

Primary source—original report or article written by the investigator who conducted the study

Problem statement—written statement that identifies the area and population to be studied and the variables involved

Proposition—statement that further clarifies the relationship between two concepts

Psychometric properties—reliability and validity of an instrument

Qualitative research — study that uses concepts that are analyzed as words to identify the relationships among variables

Quantitative research — study that uses variables that are analyzed as numbers

Random — having the characteristic of relating or belonging to a group in which each element of the population has an equal and independent chance of being chosen for the sample

Reductionism — philosophical view that an individual is no more than the sum of his or her parts and those parts can be studied separately

Research — systematic inquiry undertaken to solve problems, answer questions, or generate new knowledge

Research report — means of communicating the findings and other important aspects of a study

Sampling interval — distance, usually expressed as a number, between the elements chosen for a sample

Secondary source — description of a research study written by someone other than the investigator who conducted the study

Statistical significance — usefulness of a study's findings based on rejection of the null hypothesis and on the probability that differences between groups do not result from chance

Theoretical definition — general, abstract meaning that the researcher ascribes to a variable

Theory — formal set of interrelated concepts and propositions used to describe, explain, predict, or understand an aspect of reality

Thesis — formal research study written by a candidate for a master's degree

True score — most accurate value obtainable if the instrument were perfect

Variable — characteristic of a person or object that differs among members of the population

Vulnerable subject — any individual whose rights are at high risk of violation during a research study; vulnerable populations include children and those who are mentally impaired, terminally ill, or institutionalized

B: Answers to Study Questions

CHAPTER 1

1. The primary goal of nursing research is to develop a specialized, scientifically based body of knowledge.

2. Basic research is done to advance the body of knowledge, whereas applied research is done to remedy a particular problem.

3. Florence Nightingale furthered nursing research by emphasizing the importance of systematic observation, data collection, environmental factors, and statistical analyses.

4. A researcher might conduct a pilot study to minimize the possibility of having significant difficulties with the major study.

5. All nurses need to critique previously conducted and newly proposed research.

CHAPTER 2

1. Experimental studies noted for unethical treatment of human subjects include Nazi medical experiments, the Tuskegee syphilis study, the Jewish Chronic Disease Hospital study, and the Willowbrook hepatitis study.

2. The Nuremburg Code resulted from the unethical experimentation spotlighted during the Nazi criminal trials.

3. The three ethical principles relevant to research are respect, beneficence, and justice.

4. Human rights requiring protection are self-determination, privacy, anonymity and confidentiality, fair treatment, and protection from harm.

CHAPTER 3

1. Identification of the research problem is important because it provides direction for the entire study.

2. Nursing practice, literature, theory, and interactions with peers and researchers might be sources for research problems.

3. Factors to be considered when selecting a research problem are its significance, researchability, feasibility, and interest to the researcher.

4. A problem statement may be interrogative or declarative.

CHAPTER 4

1. A literature review is done to lay the foundation for the research or to compare and contrast the literature with the findings from the current study.

2. A review may help the researcher to identify or refine the problem, strengthen the rationale for the research, develop a conceptual framework, provide a useful approach to conducting the study, and explain or support the findings.

3. The researcher reviews research findings, theoretical information, methodological information, opinion articles, and anecdotal descriptions.

4. Indexes are the researcher's main source for manually locating articles published in journals.

5. A computer search is more current and less time-consuming than a manual search; it also allows concepts to be combined in the search.

CHAPTER 5

1. Nursing researchers are particularly interested in the key concepts of person, environment, health, and nursing.

2. A schematic model uses boxes and arrows; a mathematical model uses letters, numbers, and mathematical symbols.

3. Conceptual frameworks are based on specific concepts and propositions; theoretical frameworks are based on a theory.

4. Nursing theories used to guide nursing research include Roy's "Adaptation Model," Orem's "Self-Care Model," Rogers's "Science of Unitary Human Beings," and Neuman's "Health-Care Systems Model."

5. Theories borrowed from other disciplines used to guide nursing research include Bandura's "Social Learning Theory," Lazarus's and Selye's stress theories, Spielberger's anxiety theory, and Melzack's and Wall's pain theory.

6. Common problems related to conceptual and theoretical frameworks include use of an inappropriate or unidentified framework, use of a framework that is disconnected from the study, and use of multiple frameworks within the same study.

CHAPTER 6

1. A variable is a concept examined in a research study; a hypothesis predicts the relationship between the variables.

2. The theoretical definition of a variable is broad and abstract and is derived from literature; the operational definition reflects the procedures that the researcher performs to measure the variable.

3. The independent variable is the presumed cause and is manipulated by the researcher to examine the effect on the dependent variable.

4. A researcher would use a complex hypothesis to predict a relationship among two or more independent variables and two or more dependent variables.

5. Research questions guiding qualitative studies are usually broader and more abstract than those in quantitative research.

CHAPTER 7

1. Quantitative research is based on reductionism and uses variables that are analyzed as numbers; qualitative research is based on holism and uses concepts that are analyzed as words.

2. Threats to internal validity include history, maturation, testing, instrumentation, mortality or attrition, and selection bias.

3. The characteristics of a true experimental design are manipulation, control, and randomization.

4. The six major categories of a qualitative research design are phenomenological, grounded theory, ethnographic, historical, philosophical inquiry, and critical social theory.

5. Cross-sectional research designs involve collecting data from different subjects at one time; longitudinal research designs involve collecting data from the same subjects over time.

6. The data collection methods used in survey research designs include face-to-face interviews, telephone interviews, and written questionnaires.

7. A methodological research design involves the development, testing, and evaluation of research instruments.

CHAPTER 8

1. A population is an entire group of elements that meets the eligibility criteria and may consist of people, animals, objects, words, or events.

2. Probability sampling techniques involve selecting elements from the population using random procedures; nonprobability sampling techniques use nonrandom procedures.

3. Four types of probability sampling are simple random, stratified random, cluster, and systematic.

4. Four types of nonprobability sampling are accidental, quota, purposive, and network.

CHAPTER 9

1. Stability, internal consistency, and equivalence are three types of reliability.

2. Content, concurrent, predictive, and construct are four types of validity.

3. The levels of measurement, from lowest to highest, are nominal, ordinal, interval, and ratio.

4. Questionnaires and interviews are the most commonly used data collection methods.

5. The main disadvantage of questionnaires is the possibility of a low response rate.

6. The main advantage of a scale is its efficiency in measuring quantitatively the degree or magnitude of a variable.

7. The main advantage of physiological data collection measures is that they are objective and tend to be accurate.

CHAPTER 10

1. The purpose of data analysis is to impose order on voluminous data so that conclusions can be drawn.

2. Quantitative data analysis uses numbers and statistical computations.

3. Qualitative data analysis uses words and analytical reasoning.

4. The four categories of descriptive statistics are frequency distribution, measures of central tendency, measures of variability, and bivariate statistics.

5. Methods used to analyze qualitative data include the constant comparative method, content analysis, analytical induction, and hermeneutical analysis.

CHAPTER 11

1. The researcher uses introspection, logic, and intuition to interpret the findings.

2. Statistical significance means that any differences between groups are probably not due to chance; clinical significance means that the findings may be useful in a clinical setting.

3. Nursing implications provide practical suggestions for implementing research findings in practice.

4. The research findings might be communicated in an oral report, a poster presentation, or a written report.

5. The practicing nurse might increase research use by critically reading research literature, attending professional meetings, collaborating with nursing researchers, and participating in utilization projects.

Selected References

Brink, P.J., and Wood, M.J. *Basic Steps in Planning Research from Questions to Proposal*, 4th ed. Boston: Jones & Bartlett, 1994.

Brockopp, D.Y., and Hastings-Tolsma, M.T. *Fundamentals of Nursing Research*. Glenview, Ill.: Scott, Foresman, 1989.

Burns, N., and Grove, S.K. *The Practice of Nursing Research: Conduct, Critique and Utilization*, 2nd ed. Philadelphia: W.B. Saunders Co., 1993.

Crabtree, B.F., and Miller, W.L., eds. *Doing Qualitative Research*. Newbury Park, Calif.: Sage Publications, 1992.

Dempsey, P.A., and Dempsey, A.D. *Nursing Research with Basic Statistical Applications*, 3rd ed. Boston: Jones and Bartlett, 1992.

LoBiondo-Wood, G., and Haber, J., eds. *Nursing Research: Critical Appraisal and Utilization*, 3rd ed. St. Louis: C.V. Mosby Co., 1994.

Mateo, M.A., and Kirchhoff, K.T. *Conducting and Using Nursing Research in the Clinical Setting*. Baltimore: Williams & Wilkins Co., 1991.

Munhall, P.L., and Boyd, C.O., eds. *Nursing Research: A Qualitative Perspective*, 2nd ed. New York: National League for Nursing Press, 1993.

Nieswiadomy, R.M. *Foundations of Nursing Research*, 2nd ed. Norwalk, Conn.: Appleton & Lange, 1993.

Polit, D.F., and Hungler, B.P. *Essentials of Nursing Research: Methods, Appraisal, and Utilization*, 3rd ed. Philadelphia: J.B. Lippincott Co., 1993.

Polit, D.F., and Hungler, B.P. *Nursing Research: Principles and Methods*, 4th ed. Philadelphia: J.B. Lippincott Co., 1991.

Roberts, C.A., and Burke, S.O. *Nursing Research: A Quantitative and Qualitative Approach*. Boston: Jones and Bartlett, 1989.

Wilson, H.S. *Introducing Research in Nursing*, 2nd ed. Menlo Park, Calif.: Addison-Wesley Publishing Co., 1993.

Wilson, H.S. *Research in Nursing*, 2nd ed. Redwood City, Calif.: Addison-Wesley Health Sciences, 1989.

Index

---

t refers to a table.